HEMATOLOGY AND URINALYSIS

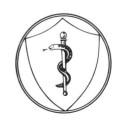

An AVI Series
AVI Publishing Company

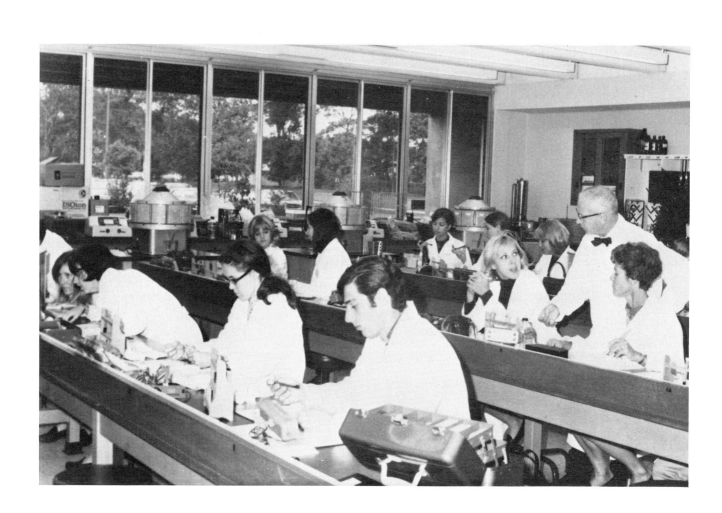

LABORATORY MANUAL OF HEMATOLOGY AND URINALYSIS

Stanley Lawrence Lamberg, B.S., M.A., M.S., Ph.D.

Registered M.T.
Professor
Department of Medical Laboratory Technology
State University of New York
Agricultural and Technical College
Farmingdale, New York

Robert Rothstein, B.A., M.A.

Registered M.T.
Chairman
Division of Human Services
Professor
Department of Medical Laboratory Technology
State University of New York
Agricultural and Technical College
Farmingdale, New York

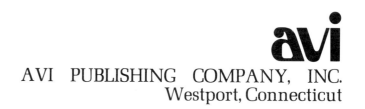

AVI PUBLISHING COMPANY, INC.
Westport, Connecticut

ISBN-0-87055-268-6

Printed in the United States of America

Preface

This laboratory manual is written primarily for the beginning student in Medical Technology. The aim of this manual is to introduce the student to some of the basic hematological and urinalysis tests commonly performed in the clinical laboratory. Although the emphasis is on the performance of the techniques, the theoretical aspects of the tests are discussed as well as the reasons why the steps of a procedure are carried out as described. All procedures are first described by manual methods, and in later exercises automated methodologies are presented.

In learning manual methods, repetition of the procedures is an important requirement in development of technique. Thus, the more one practices the methods correctly, the more proficient in terms of speed and accuracy one will become. In this manner, the student will develop confidence in performance capabilities. On the job this sense of confidence is reassuring to the patient and helps to relieve the patient's apprehension. By careful use of this manual by the student and the instructor, and with repetition of the procedures, the student can become quite competent in doing a complete blood count, ancillary tests and basic urine examinations.

Since hematologic tests and a urinalysis are performed as routine diagnostic or screening tests, it is imperative that the student of Medical Technology be thoroughly familiar with the procedures in this manual. More sophisticated diagnostic procedures are discussed in the other manuals of the *Functional Medical Laboratory Technology* series. For example, immunohematology, a special branch of hematology, is the study of the blood group systems (such as ABO, Rh, etc.). This topic is covered in the *Laboratory Manual of Serology, Immunology and Blood Banking*.

All medical laboratory technologists must perform all tests in an exacting manner and with highest accuracy since the results submitted are relied upon by the physician in the diagnosis and prognosis of disease and charting a course of treatment.

This laboratory manual attempts to instill in the student the sense of professionalism and accuracy inherent in the work of allied health personnel while gaining proficiency in the actual test procedures.

The authors wish to express their appreciation to Adele Traurig for preliminary typing and to Marsha Mason for the final typing of the manuscript.

John W. Frost gave much of his time and talent to the final illustrations and Joanne Christiansen contributed some preliminary sketches.

The members of the Department of Medical Laboratory Technology at the State University of New York at Farmingdale, despite their busy schedules, gave freely of their time.

Finally, the authors would like to acknowledge the interest and encouragement of Dr. George G. Cook and Dr. Donald K. Tressler, AVI Publishing Co., and Barbara Flouton and Arlene Hoeppner of the AVI editorial department for their assistance in bringing this manual into being.

STANLEY LAWRENCE LAMBERG
ROBERT ROTHSTEIN

December 1977

Contents

General Considerations, Methods of Blood Collection, Coagulation and Bleeding Time

I. COMPOSITION OF THE BLOOD

Blood is a specialized form of connective tissue. It consists of the formed elements, made up of white cells, red cells, platelets, and a fluid substance, the plasma.

A. Formed Elements

The formed elements are in a ratio of

erythrocyte (RBC) : leukocyte (WBC) : platelet (thrombocyte)
  500   :   1   :   30

In terms of size, the leukocytes are the largest, erythrocytes smaller, and the platelets the smallest.

B. Plasma

The plasma is the intercellular fluid in which the formed elements are suspended as well as solute molecules dissolved. The major component of the plasma is water. Within the plasma true solutes are dissolved and colloids are permanently suspended. Examples of true solutes are nutritive substances from the digestive process, salts, vitamins, end-products of metabolism and hormones. Examples of colloids are blood proteins, blood coagulation factors, enzymes and antibodies.

C. Serum

When blood coagulates, fibrinogen precipitates as a network of fibrin strands. As the clot retracts, a clear, yellow fluid exudes from the clot; this fluid is serum. The major chemical difference between plasma and serum is that serum lacks fibrinogen, while plasma contains fibrinogen.

D. Volume of Blood

The average adult has about 5 liters of blood, approximately 3 liters plasma to 2 liters formed elements, or 60% fluid to 40% formed elements ratio.

E. pH of the Blood

pH of the blood is 7.35–7.45, average value 7.4.

F. Specific Gravity of the Blood

$$\text{specific gravity} \quad = \quad \frac{\text{weight of a volume of blood at 4°C}}{\text{weight of the same volume of distilled water at 4°C}}$$

Specific gravity blood = 1.048–1.066
Specific gravity serum = 1.026–1.031, since fibrinogen and formed elements are removed.

II.   COMPLETE BLOOD COUNT (CBC)

During the laboratory sessions, the most frequently requested hematological tests in the clinical laboratory will be performed. The hematological tests, which are mainly concerned with the cellular elements of the blood, are distinguished from the broader and more general term of "blood tests."

The basic complete blood count (CBC) usually includes: hemoglobin estimation (Hgb or Hb), white cell count (WBC), red cell count (RBC), differential white cell count (differential or diff). Some laboratories also include the hematocrit, platelet count, reticulocyte count, mean cell volume, red cell indexes, stained red cell examination, coagulation time, etc., in a CBC.

The results of the tests are reported on a hematology form of which there are many types. The report should include the hospital's name, patient's name, identification (I.D.) number, room, date, tests requested and physician who is requesting the tests.

The results in the report are extremely confidential and are a matter of concern between the technician and physician. The test results are reported to the physician, never to the patient, unless specifically authorized by the physician.

III.   COLLECTION OF THE BLOOD SAMPLE

In order to perform a complete blood count, blood must be collected either by A. fingertip puncture or B. venipuncture. The basis of hematological testing depends on the proper collection of the blood sample in order to obtain reliable results.

A. Fingertip Puncture

The fingertip puncture is used when small quantities of blood are to be examined for hemoglobin estimation, RBC, WBC, platelet counts, blood smears and a few other tests.

The fingertip is the preferred site of collection of small volumes of blood, since the patient observing the procedure becomes less apprehensive. Other sites of blood collection where this technique is applicable are the earlobe, heel, or big toe of infants.

The site of blood collection must be warm to ensure free flow of blood, otherwise, the blood sample will not be truly representative of the blood in the vascular system.

1. **Assembly of Apparatus on Blood Tray.**—The apparatus for basic fingertip puncture and collection of blood is placed on the blood tray. The blood tray is filled with these basic items before the technician leaves the laboratory to make the collections. There are many varieties of blood trays commercially available.

The blood tray should contain adequate amounts of the following equipment for the <u>basic</u> fingertip puncture.

a. Hematology requisition slips as noted above
b. 70% Alcohol (70% alcohol is used as the disinfectant, since this percentage kills the vegetative and spore forms of bacteria within less than 1 min)
c. Sterile gauze pads, cotton or alcohol swabs
d. Sterile disposable blood lancets
e. Aspirator (mouthpiece and rubber tubing)
f. Clean, dry, nonchipped blood pipettes

   (1) Hemoglobin pipettes (aspirator should be attached to Hb pipette before starting the procedure as blood for this test is collected first)
   (2) White cell pipettes
   (3) Red cell pipettes

g. Glass slides (3″ × 1″)
h. Blood diluting fluids

   (1) Hemoglobin diluting fluid—Drabkin's solution (rack with test tubes should be carried in tray)
   (2) White cell diluting fluid—2% acetic acid or 1% (0.1N) HCl
   (3) Red cell diluting fluid—Hayem's solution (or others employed by some laboratories)

i. Pencil, small pad of paper

If additional hematological tests are requested, fill tray with necessary items.

Place apparatus within easy reach on clean toweling. Loosen lids from diluting fluid bottles before you start so as not to waste time when diluting the blood, otherwise the blood may clot during taking of the sample. Wash your hands before beginning the procedure.

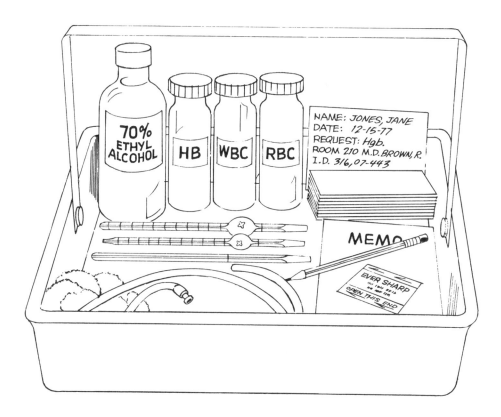

FIG. 1.1.   BLOOD TRAY FOR FINGERTIP PUNCTURE

2.   Preparation of the Finger.—

a.   The puncture is made on the third finger of the hand. Vigorously massage the finger from base to tip 5 or 6 times with thumb and index finger of one hand. Hold patient's fingertip with thumb and index finger of other hand (see Fig. 1.2).

b.   Alcohol swab the ball of the finger with 70% alcohol; allow to air dry.

c.   With a piece of <u>dry</u>, sterile gauze or cotton, <u>thoroughly dry the ball of the finger</u>. If finger is not dry, the blood will not form <u>a rounded drop and will run down the sides</u>.

3.   Puncturing the Finger.—A separate disposable sterile blood lancet is used for each patient to prevent spread of the virus of serum hepatitis. The lancet is used once and thrown away after use.

Puncture the patient <u>deeply</u> the first time to avoid repeated punctures. The ball of the finger is punctured with a quick drop and quick rise of the lancet (see Fig. 1.3).

a.   Unwrap the lancet; firmly grasp lancet in one hand. Hold patient's finger firmly at first joint with your other hand. You may wish to have patient's head turned to the side so as not to observe the actual puncture (and reassure the patient by saying, "This won't hurt much.").

b. With a rapid puncture, stab deeply into the ball of the finger.

c. Observe the instructor puncturing the finger.

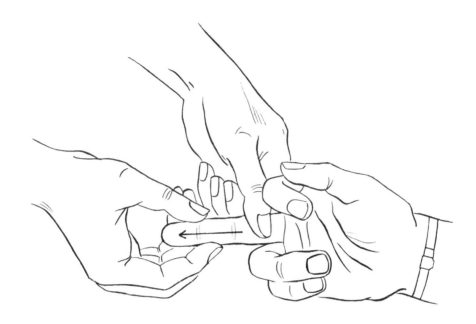

FIG. 1.2.   MASSAGING THE FINGER

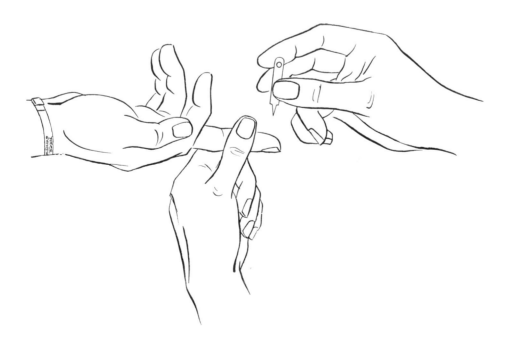

FIG. 1.3.   USE OF LANCET FOR FINGER PUNCTURE

4. **Eliminating the First Drop of Blood.**—The first drop of blood is not a true sample of the patient's blood, since it contains lymph or tissue fluid and extraneous matter clinging to the surface of the skin. The first drop is wiped away and the area is wiped dry with a piece of sterile gauze or cotton. If ball of finger is not dry, the next drop will not form a rounded drop.

5. **Production of Second Large, Rounded Drop of Blood.**—

   a. A second large, rounded drop of blood is produced at the site of the puncture by massaging the patient's finger several times toward tip of finger.

   b. You may also squeeze <u>gently</u> on the sides of the finger near the puncture site with both thumbs. If you squeeze too hard, lymph flows out and you will not have a representative sample of blood.

   c. After the last massage, clamp down hard at the first joint of the patient's finger. This action dams the blood off, allows the blood to well up in the fingertip and to flow out of the puncture to form a large, rounded drop.

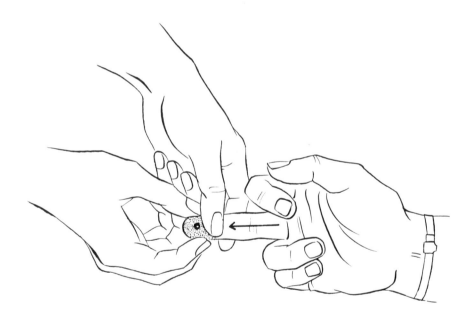

FIG. 1.4.   PRODUCING A SECOND, LARGE ROUNDED DROP OF BLOOD

An alternative method may also be used. Swab finger with the alcohol, remove sterile lancet, puncture finger while still wet with alcohol. Then dry finger with sterile swab, squeeze finger gently and wipe away first 2 drops of blood.

6. **Withdrawal of the Blood.**—The technique of withdrawal of fingertip blood into the pipette is as follows (see Fig. 1.5).

   a. Attach aspirator to pipette.

   b. Hold pipette so as not to cover the markings.

c. Brace fingers, holding pipette on patient's finger. This enables the technician to move with patient's movement and keeps tip of pipette in the drop of blood.

d. Hold tip of pipette loosely in drop of blood so as not to touch the skin, and withdraw required quantities. If tip of pipette is pressed against puncture, blood will stop flowing into the pipette.

e. The blood is then diluted to perform hemoglobin estimation, total red cell and white cell counts.

f. Blood is also withdrawn for the blood smear for the differential white cell count.

The details of performing the basic tests of the complete blood count will be described in later exercises.

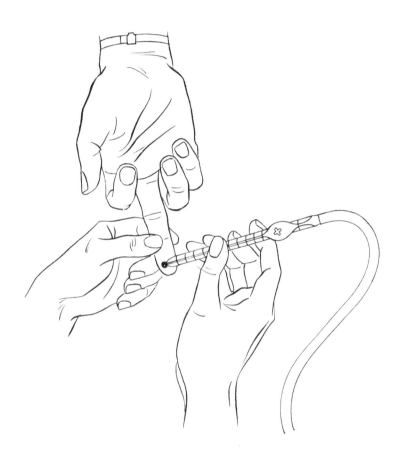

FIG. 1.5.   COLLECTION OF BLOOD FROM A FINGERTIP PUNCTURE

7.   **Preventing Further Bleeding.—**

a. Place an alcohol swab on the puncture.

b. Ask patient to hold the swab on the puncture until it stops bleeding.

c. Thank the patient for being so cooperative.

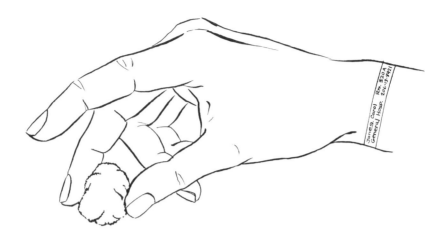

FIG. 1.6. PATIENT HOLDING SWAB TO STOP BLEEDING

8. **Labeling the Specimens.**—To prevent loss of fluid from pipette after blood has been diluted, keep pipettes in a horizontal position. (Most hematological trays have racks to accomplish this.)

   a. An alternative method would be to label collected specimens with patient's name, I.D. number, room, etc., on a piece of paper. Push pipettes through the paper pointed end first; keep pipettes in a horizontal position. This also keeps tips of pipettes from touching anything, otherwise fluid may drain out. (Pipette closures of various types may also be used.) (See Fig. 1.7).
   b. After blood smear has dried, write patient's name on the slide in pencil.
   c. Place the labeled specimens safely on the blood tray.
   d. Clean up area and put apparatus away.

B. Venipuncture

When a large quantity of blood is necessary, blood is obtained from a vein. The superficial veins of the extremities are ideal sites for venipuncture. Blood can be obtained from several superficial veins, such as the median cubital in the bend of the elbow, dorsal hand veins, wrist or ankle veins. The median cubital vein is most frequently used because veins of the forearm are larger than the other mentioned veins.

The venipuncture is performed either by a syringe or vacutainer (Becton–Dickinson Co.). Vacutainers have the advantage in that they are a disposable, sterile apparatus, eliminating the hazard of serum hepatitis transmission.

1. **Assembly of Apparatus on the Blood Tray.**—The apparatus necessary for the venipuncture is assembled on the blood tray.

   a. Hematology requisition slip with patient's name, I.D. number, room, date, physician's name, tests requested, etc.

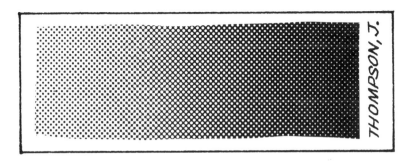

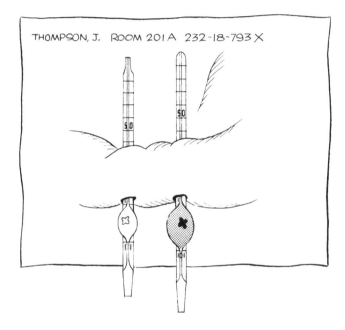

FIG. 1.7.   A METHOD OF IDENTIFYING PATIENTS' BLOOD SAMPLES

b. 70% Alcohol

c. Sterile gauze pads, cotton or alcohol swabs

d. Tourniquet

e. Sterile needles (20 to 22 gauge). Size of needle varies with size of vein from which blood is to be withdrawn.

f. Syringe with matching numbered barrel and plunger. Size of syringe varies with amount of blood to be withdrawn.

g. Plain and anticoagulated, stoppered test tubes

Or, in lieu of e, f, and g

h. Vacutainer consisting of

(1) Plain or anticoagulated rubber-stoppered evacuated tubes

(2) Plastic holder

(3) Disposable double-pointed needles

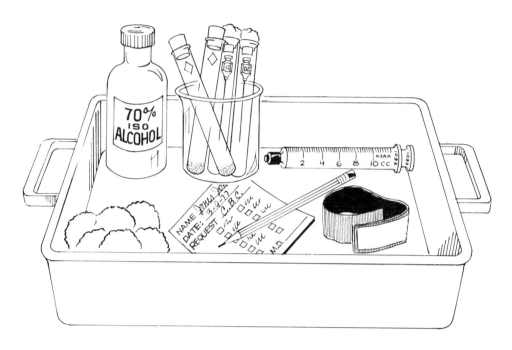

FIG. 1.8.   PHLEBOTOMY TRAY

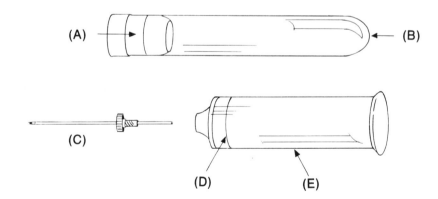

FIG. 1.9.   DESCRIPTION OF PARTS OF VACUTAINER
(A) Rubber stopper.   (D) Guide line.
(B) Glass tube.   (E) Plastic holder.
(C) Double-pointed needle.

Color-coded rubber stoppers indicate if vacutainer tube is plain or has a type of anticoagulant in the tube.

i.   Test tube rack to hold tubes
j.   Wax pencil and labels to label collected blood samples
k.   Bottle of smelling salts in case patient faints

2.   Identifying the Patient.—

    a.   Compare the name of patient, I.D. number, room and physician's name on requisition form with name on identification wrist band to be sure you have correct patient.

    b.   After the blood is collected, label tubes in which blood is to be collected with patient's name, I.D. number, room, physician's name and tests to be performed on the blood.

3.   Positioning the Patient.—

    a.   Have the patient assume a comfortable position, either lying down or sitting. Place blood tray on a nearby table where it cannot be upset by movements of the patient.

    b.   Make any adjustments of the furniture to enable you to work with free action.

    c.   If the patient is in bed, move patient to edge of the bed (if possible) and have patient's arm extended.

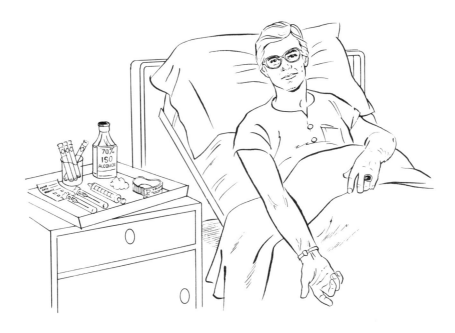

FIG. 1.10.   POSITION OF BED PATIENT FOR PHLEBOTOMY

       If patient is ambulatory, sit patient alongside of a table on which arm can be extended. Support arm under elbow to keep arm extended.

    d.   Technician should sit or stand opposite the patient, whichever is more comfortable to give the technician a good command of the situation.

    e.   Never have the patient standing or sitting on a high stool, in case patient faints. If patient does faint, render appropriate first aid.

    f.   While the above adjustments are being made, the patient should be reassured to relieve apprehension. (A good sense of humor goes a long way.)

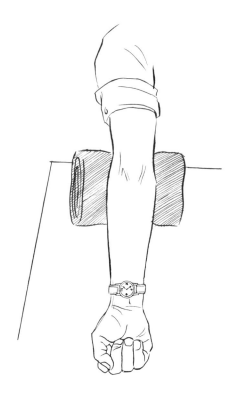

FIG. 1.11.   POSITION OF AMBULATORY PATIENT FOR PHLEBOTOMY

4. **Applying the Tourniquet.**—The tourniquet should be applied before preparation of syringe or vacutainer, which takes only seconds. A piece of rubber tubing can serve as a tourniquet. More recently, the Velket tourniquet is used. This is a band of gum rubber, which is easily and quickly applied without making any ties. The tourniquet of sufficient tension is placed above the bend in the elbow in the prescribed manner to enlarge the veins of forearm. (One will learn with experience the degree of tension required.) The tourniquet is applied to block off venous circulation. The patient is instructed to open and close the fist to build up blood pressure; as a result, the forearm veins become more prominent (see Fig. 1.12).

5. **Preparing Needle and Syringe or Vacutainer.**—

    a. If sterile needle and syringe are used, the needle is seated on end of syringe by inverting test tube containing sterile needle over end of syringe so needle slips onto end of syringe. Seat needle firmly on end of syringe. Check to see if needle is clogged by moving plunger up and down forcing air through the needle. With needle attached to syringe, insert needle into test tube to keep it sterile. (*NOTE:* Some syringes are equipped with Luer locks.) (See Fig. 1.13).

    b. If vacutainer is used, thread sterile disposable double-pointed needle into plastic holder. Place vacutainer tube in holder with rear end of needle touching stopper. The vacutainer tube is pushed forward until top of stopper is level with guide line on holder. In this position, the rear end of the double-pointed needle is embedded in the rubber stopper, but the vacuum has not been broken. Keep front end of needle in plastic container to maintain sterility (see Fig. 1.14).

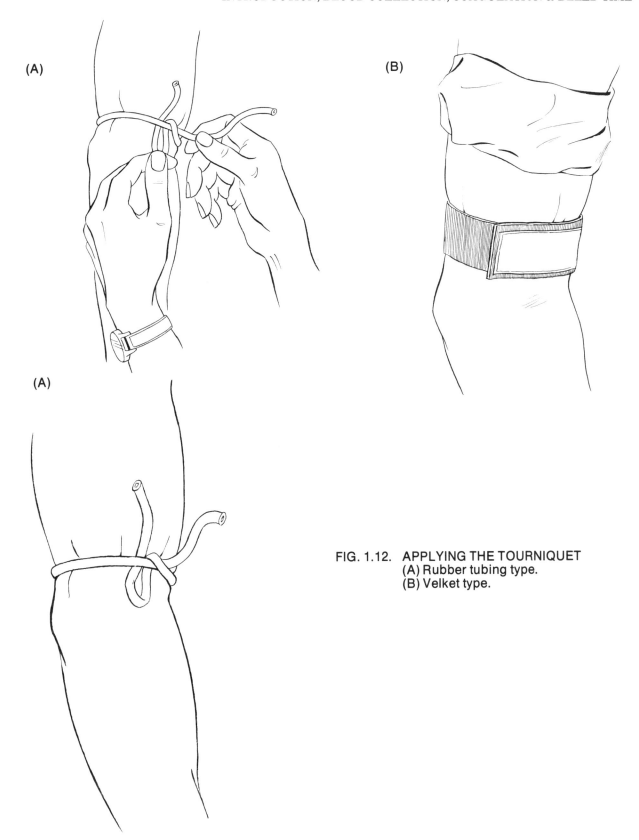

(A)

(A)

(B)

FIG. 1.12.   APPLYING THE TOURNIQUET
(A) Rubber tubing type.
(B) Velket type.

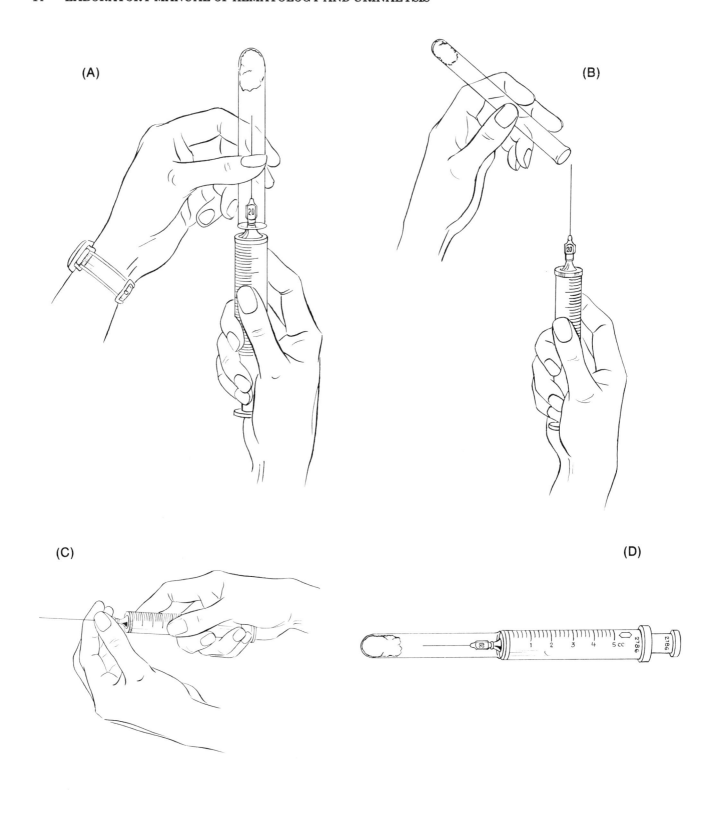

FIG. 1.13.   METHOD OF ATTACHING STERILE NEEDLE TO STERILE SYRINGE
(A) Dropping needle from tube onto syringe.   (C) Locking needle onto syringe.
(B) Needle on syringe.   (D) Syringe and needle ready for use.

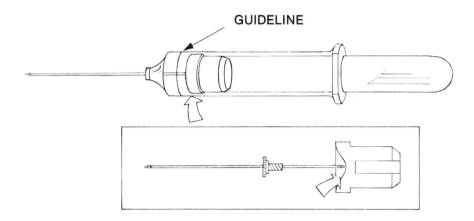

FIG. 1.14. POSITION OF STERILE DOUBLE-POINTED NEEDLE BEFORE VACUUM IS BROKEN

6.   Selecting the Vein.—

a. If the veins are visible, choose the most prominent one and, with your finger, trace the path of the vein.

b. If veins are not visible, palpate the area with your finger; the veins will reveal themselves as elastic-like tubes beneath the surface of the skin. With your finger, trace the path of a vein.

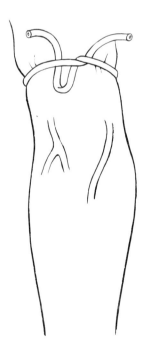

FIG. 1.15. VEINS OF THE FOREARM WITH APPLIED TOURNIQUET

c. If veins are difficult to locate, proceed as follows.

(1) Continue to have the patient open and close the fist.
(2) Apply heavy massaging action on the lower part of extremity and moving toward the elbow.
(3) Slap the area several times to make veins more prominent.
(4) Palpate area to feel for a vein; trace path of vein with your finger.

d. If veins in one arm cannot be located, apply tourniquet to other arm and inspect the veins. If veins in bend of elbow cannot be located, use the veins in other parts of extremities.

Veins are sometimes more difficult to palpate in obese people and children. If the technician is having difficulty in locating a vein or performing the entire procedure, ask for help from others. Some hospitals employ technician phlebotomists who specialize solely in drawing blood.

7.   Applying the Antiseptic.—

a. Thoroughly cleanse the area of the puncture with an alcohol swab (gauze pad or cotton ball moistened with 70% alcohol). You may palpate the area again, but afterward cleanse again with an alcohol swab.

b. Lay a fresh alcohol swab in a convenient place as it will be used later in the procedure.

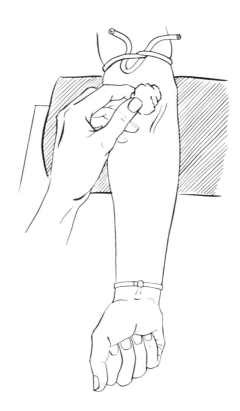

FIG. 1.16. APPLYING ALCOHOL BEFORE VENIPUNCTURE

8.   Inserting the Needle.—

a. Hold syringe in one hand. If syringe is used, the heel of the hand holds plunger down in the barrel to prevent air from entering the syringe. The index finger is placed alongside of the hub of the needle to guide the needle.

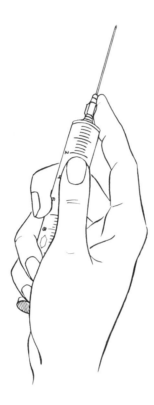

FIG. 1.17.   CORRECT WAY OF HOLDING THE SYRINGE

b. A proposed point of entry is selected. This point should be at the thickest portion of the vein. Enter the vein below the proposed point to prevent going past the vein.

c. To prevent veins from rolling beneath the skin as the needle approaches, fix the vein in position by pressing down firmly with the thumb and first finger (of hand not holding the syringe or vacutainer) above and below proposed point of entry, and pull the skin taut.

d. Point the needle in same direction the vein is running. Hold syringe or vacutainer at 15° angle with patient's arm with the needle's bevel edge up. The position of the needle's bevel depends on technician's preference. Some technicians like bevel up, since they feel this helps "steer the needle." Without hesitation, push the needle firmly and deliberately through the skin into the vein. As the needle enters the vein, a little "give" may be felt.

(A)   (B)

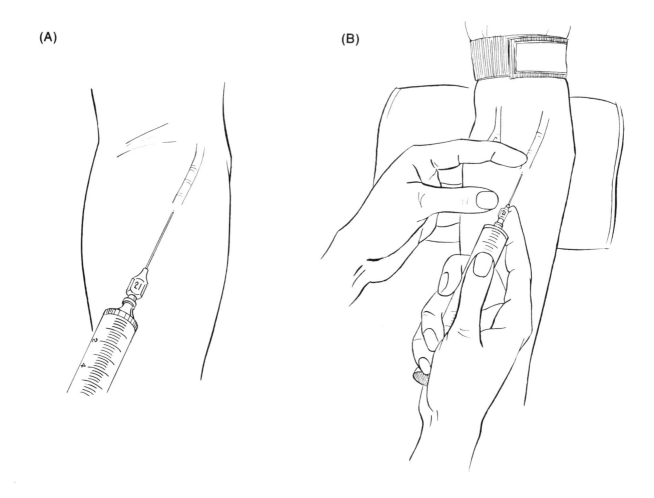

FIG. 1.18.   (A) POINTING NEEDLE FOR VENIPUNCTURE
(B) PROPOSED SITE OF NEEDLE ENTRY AND HOLDING VEIN IN PLACE

The needle is held in line with the vein to keep pressure on vein downward, so that on entering the vein, the vein will not roll sideways. Furthermore, the needle entering the vein from above has a larger area for penetration.

The proper angle of syringe or vacutainer is necessary, for if the angle is too great, the needle will go through the vein. If the angle is too small, the needle either will be on top of the vein's wall or only penetrate the wall without reaching the lumen of the vein (see Fig. 1.19).

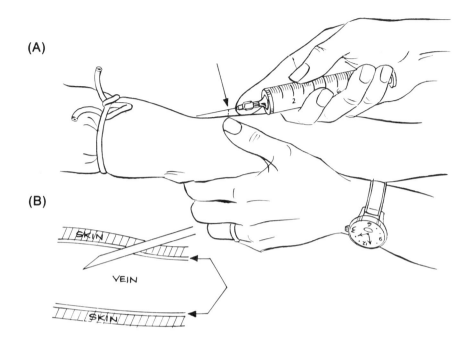

FIG. 1.19. (A) PROPER ANGLE FOR NEEDLE INSERTION
(B) MAGNIFIED VIEW OF NEEDLE ENTRY

9.   Withdrawal of the Blood.—

a. With the Syringe.—

(1)   If the needle is correctly in the vein, pull plunger slowly back with the hand not holding the syringe. If plunger sticks, twist it as you pull. Keep the index finger of hand holding syringe alongside of hub of the needle and brace the finger on arm of patient. This allows you to move with patient's movements. Keep your eye on the needle to keep needle in the vein. Do not wiggle or put pressure on the needle; this pushes edge of needle against vein wall and is painful.

(2)   If the needle is not initially in vein correctly and blood does not enter syringe when plunger is pulled back, use the index finger of hand not holding the syringe to probe for needle's position. The needle could be in any of the three following locations:

(a)   Needle has not penetrated vein wall into lumen. Fix the vein and push needle in farther.

(b)   Needle is to the side of the vein. Draw needle back slightly, fix the vein and redirect needle into vein.

(c)   Needle has penetrated completely through the vein. Fix vein, slowly withdraw needle and simultaneously pull back the plunger. This action allows you to observe the appearance of blood when needle is correctly in the lumen of the vein.

If you are unable to enter the vein, release tourniquet, completely withdraw the needle, apply an alcohol swab and have patient bend arm up. Make another venipuncture on the same or other arm of patient.

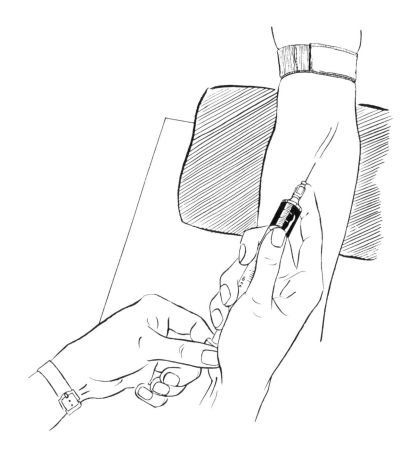

FIG. 1.20.   DRAWING BLOOD INTO SYRINGE

(3)   If needle is initially in lumen of vein and blood collection starts and then stops, three factors can be cited for this problem.

(a)   Bevel of needle is pressing against vein wall and no blood can enter the needle. Very gently wiggle needle and pull back on plunger.

(b)   Needle may have slipped out of vein. If so, determine position of needle point with index finger of hand not holding the syringe, fix vein and reinsert needle.

(c)   Needle may have gone through the vein. Withdraw needle until point is back in vein and simultaneously slowly pull back on plunger. Suction allows you to observe the appearance of blood when needle is again correctly positioned in vein's lumen.

If you cannot get needle into vein, release tourniquet, completely withdraw needle, apply alcohol swab. Have patient bend arm up. Transfer any blood you obtained to tube; clean needle and syringe with water. If you still need more blood, make another venipuncture with another sterile needle and syringe.

b. With the Vacutainer.—

(1)   If needle is correctly positioned in lumen of vein, push vacutainer tube forward with heel of hand that is holding the vacutainer. The rear point of the double-end needle will completely penetrate through the stopper. This will break the vacuum in the vacutainer tube and blood will flow immediately into the vacutainer.

(2)   An alternate method to break the vacuum is to hold the vacutainer as a hypodermic syringe. The plastic holder provides a finger grip for the index finger and third finger. The vacutainer tube acts as a plunger, pushed in with the thumb.

(3)   If needle is not properly inserted in vein, blood will not be drawn or be only slowly or partially drawn. Proceed as described previously (as with syringe) until venipuncture is signaled by an intake of blood into vacutainer tube.

(4)   If vein cannot be located, to maintain or preserve vacuum, remove vacutainer tube from rear needle before withdrawing needle completely from the arm.

(5)   Multiple specimens can be drawn from one venipuncture without loss of blood by releasing the tourniquet while first tube is filling and switching tubes while needle remains in the vein. The rear end of the needle is covered by a rubber closure that will keep blood from flowing out.

(6)   Venous collapse can be minimized by using a vacutainer adapter and smaller gauge needles to slow up flow of blood. The proper degree of vacuum in each vacutainer tube is set for the withdrawal of a specific volume of blood.

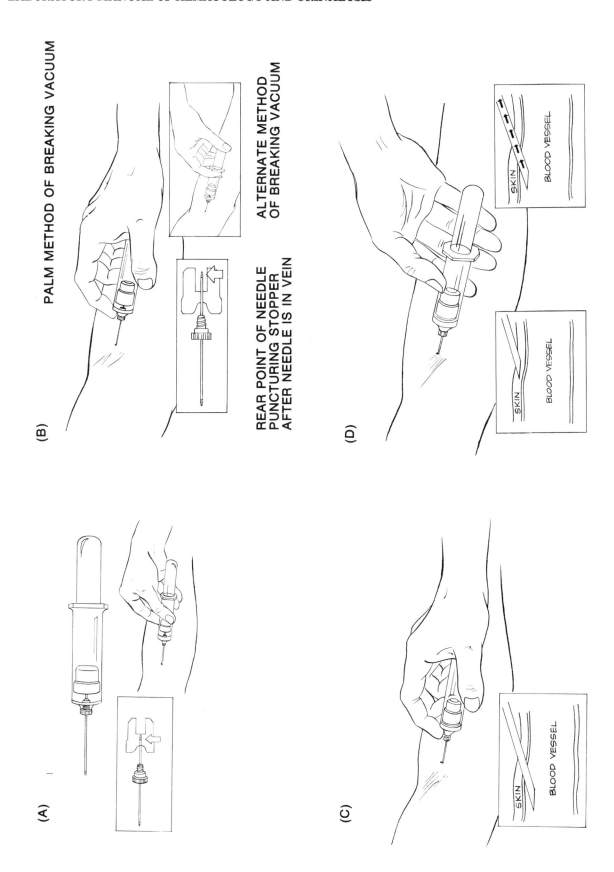

(A)

(B)

PALM METHOD OF BREAKING VACUUM

ALTERNATE METHOD
OF BREAKING VACUUM

REAR POINT OF NEEDLE
PUNCTURING STOPPER
AFTER NEEDLE IS IN VEIN

(C)

SKIN

BLOOD VESSEL

(D)

SKIN

BLOOD VESSEL

SKIN

BLOOD VESSEL

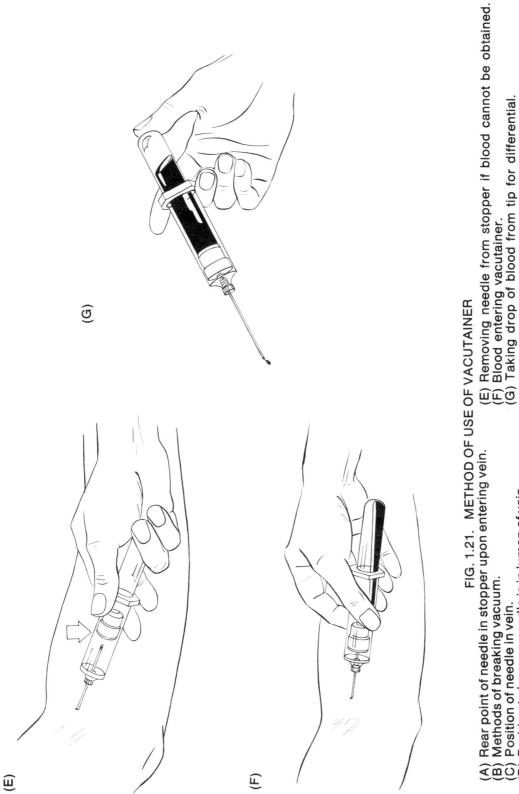

FIG. 1.21.   METHOD OF USE OF VACUTAINER

(A) Rear point of needle in stopper upon entering vein.
(B) Methods of breaking vacuum.
(C) Position of needle in vein.
(D) Probing to be sure needle is in lumen of vein.
(E) Removing needle from stopper if blood cannot be obtained.
(F) Blood entering vacutainer.
(G) Taking drop of blood from tip for differential.

10. **Withdrawal of the Tourniquet.**—When the syringe or vacutainer contains the amount of blood required for test(s), have the patient open the clenched fist. Release the tourniquet with hand not holding syringe or vacutainer. The pressure must be released before withdrawal of the needle, as blood would continue to flow from the needle hole.

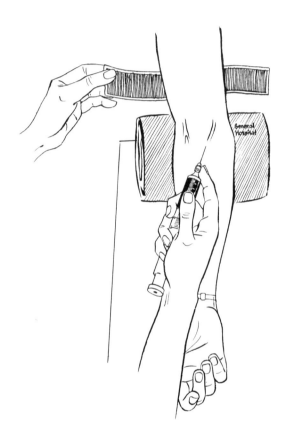

FIG. 1.22.   RELEASING TOURNIQUET BEFORE WITHDRAWAL OF NEEDLE

11. **Withdrawal of the Needle.**—

a. With hand not holding syringe or vacutainer, pick up a previously prepared alcohol swab. Without pressure, <u>gently</u> apply swab to puncture as needle is slowly withdrawn.

b. When needle is out of arm, apply <u>firm</u> pressure on the puncture. Have patient bend arm up with swab in place. Advise patient to do this for 3 to 5 min. This time period allows for blood coagulation to plug the hole in the vessel. The initial gentle pressure of the alcohol swab and the slow withdrawal of the needle is necessary to prevent injury to the vein as the needle is withdrawn.

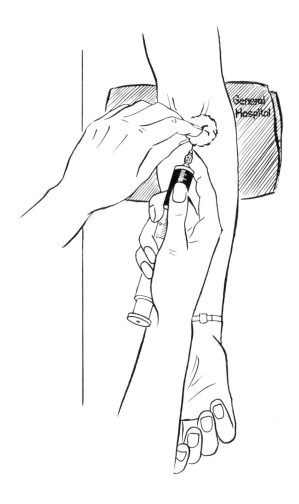

FIG. 1.23. WITHDRAWAL OF NEEDLE

12. Transferring the Blood.—

a. While patient is applying pressure to the wound, the technician transfers the blood from the syringe to the plain or anticoagulated test tubes.

b. Hold plunger of syringe with little finger of one hand; remove needle from the syringe. This allows transfer of blood without injury to the blood cells, since forcing the blood cells through small bore of needle with force of the plunger would cause blood cells to break. Transfer blood to the correct test tubes. Hold syringe so blood flows down side walls of test tube rather than down the center.

c. Stopper anticoagulated tube and invert 10–12 times to mix blood with anticoagulant. Do not shake.

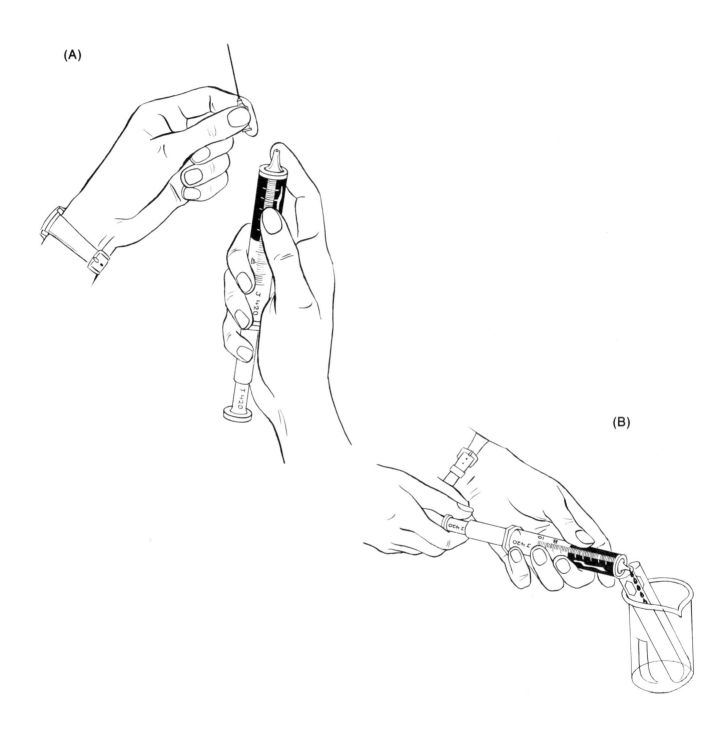

Fig. 1.24.   (A) CORRECT MANNER OF HOLDING SYRINGE FULL OF BLOOD
AND REMOVING OF THE NEEDLE
(B) PUTTING BLOOD INTO TEST TUBE

d. Blood in plain test tube—do not invert. It will clot in about 30 min. Centrifuge to produce serum for 10 min at 1000–2000 rpm.

e. If blood is collected in vacutainer tubes, invert anticoagulated tubes as above. Do nothing to plain tube.

f. The tubes should now be labeled with the patient's identification.

13. Cleaning the Non-disposable Needle and Syringe.—

a. Needle and syringe should be washed in cold tap water by flushing action.

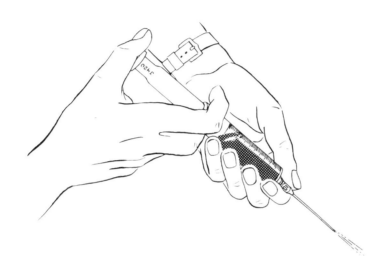

FIG. 1.25. RINSING SYRINGE AND NEEDLE

b. Separate barrel of syringe from plunger to prevent "freezing" of these two parts together.

c. If blood clogs the needle, push a stylet through the bore of the needle several times.

d. Needles and syringes can then be sterilized later before being used again. Plastic disposable syringes and disposable needles can be used to eliminate cleaning and sterilization steps. Vacutainer also has disposable equipment, completely eliminating this step.

14. Checking the Patient's Wound.—

a. After patient has applied pressure, check wound to observe if bleeding has stopped.

b. If bleeding has not stopped, continue pressure until bleeding stops.

c. If bleeding has stopped, cleanse area with a fresh alcohol swab and cover wound with a band-aid.

d. Thank the patient.

e. Clean up work area and prepare blood tray for next patient.

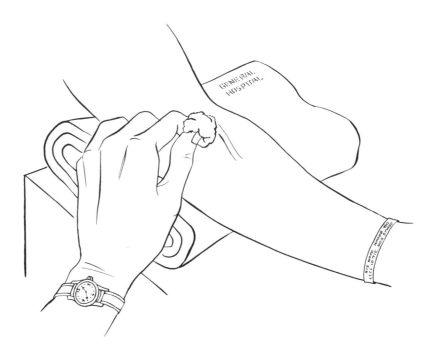

FIG. 1.26.   CHECKING SITE OF VENIPUNCTURE

IV. USE OF ANTICOAGULANTS

Anticoagulants prevent blood from coagulating by inactivating one of the essential factors in coagulation. There are several routinely used anticoagulants.

A. Mixture of Ammonium Oxalate and Potassium Oxalate

This mixture is sometimes called a double oxalate salt. The ratio of ammonium oxalate to potassium oxalate is 3:2. This anticoagulant is unsuitable for cellular examination since erythrocytes crenate, leukocytes exhibit many artifacts and platelets clump. Do not use this anticoagulant for chemical determination of nitrogen and potassium, since these elements are present in the oxalate salts. (*NOTE:* Since the double oxalate is in liquid form when prepared, the required amount of solution should be placed in tubes and thoroughly dried before blood is added.)

B. Sodium or Potassium Salts of Ethylenediaminetetraacetic Acid (EDTA)

This salt is also known as Versene or Sequestrene. It is the most widely used anticoagulant for hematological tests, since integrity of cell morphology is maintained for many hours if blood is refrigerated. The potassium salt is more soluble than the sodium salt.

C. Sodium Citrate

This anticoagulant is used mainly in collection of blood for transfusions.

The preceding three anticoagulants remove calcium ions from the blood by binding the calcium, one of the essential coagulation factors. Anticoagulants acting in this manner are called chelating agents.

D. Heparin

Heparin is a naturally occurring anticoagulant, since it is found in the body. Commercially prepared heparin is a good anticoagulant for prevention of hemolysis, but is a poor anticoagulant for examination of blood smears, since it produces a blue background in a Wright's stained or Giemsa's stained smear. Heparin acts by inhibition of thrombin formation; thus, it is an antithrombin agent.

V. HOW TO PERFORM A COMPLETE BLOOD COUNT

A. Preliminary Preparation

1. Assemble equipment as needed for either fingertip puncture or venipuncture (see Section III, A.1 and B.1 respectively).
2. Prepare patient for either fingertip puncture or venipuncture (see Section III, A.2, B.2 and B.3 respectively).
3. Blood from a fingertip puncture is collected for testing in the following order, as the largest amount of blood is collected first and smallest collected last. Since blood is flowing rapidly upon first making the puncture, a larger volume can be obtained. Blood from venipuncture can be tested in this order, also.

    a. Blood smears for the differential count
    b. Hemoglobin determination
    c. White blood cell count
    d. Red blood cell count

The performance of these tests will be described in later laboratory exercises.

4. **Preparation of the Blood.**—Before performing a complete blood count (CBC), blood has to undergo some form of preparation. This involves diluting the blood with diluting fluid and making blood smears.

B. Diluting the Blood

Since the blood cells in the sample are too highly concentrated to easily count, the blood must be diluted. The dilution is made by drawing up a measured quantity of blood and a measured quantity of diluting fluid into a pipette.

1. **Hemoglobin Determination.**—Draw up <u>exactly</u> 20 mm³ of blood in a hemoglobin pipette. To accurately pipette a measured quantity of blood, draw blood up slightly past the marking of the quantity desired. Remove pipette from the blood, hold pipette horizontally and wipe sides of pipette with a tissue. Tease blood out to the mark by touching tissue to tip of pipette and by slight blowing with your breath. Expel the blood into the hemoglobin diluting fluid. The hemoglobin diluting fluids are Drabkin's solution, 1% (0.1N) HCl or 0.1N NaOH.

(A)

(B)

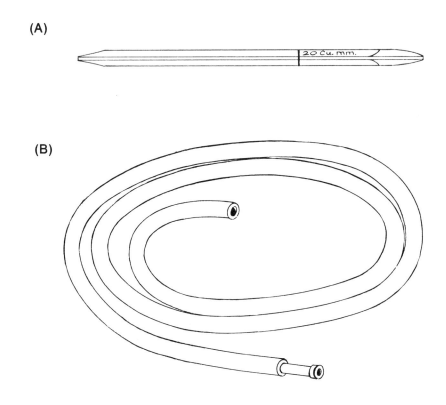

FIG. 1.27.   (A) HEMOGLOBIN PIPETTE
            (B) ASPIRATOR

Hemoglobin estimation is usually carried out colorimetrically by the Sahli or Drabkin's methods. The latter is the <u>preferred</u> and <u>recommended</u> method.

2. **White Blood Cell Count.**—Into the white blood cell pipette, draw blood to the 0.5 mark <u>exactly</u>. Then fill the pipette with white cell diluting fluid to the 11.0 mark. White cell <u>diluting</u> fluids are 0.1N HCl or 2% acetic acid. The latter is preferred (see Fig. 1.28).

3. **Red Blood Cell Count.**—In the red cell pipette, draw blood to the 0.5 mark. Then fill the pipette with red blood cell diluting fluid to the 101 mark. Red blood cell diluting fluids, as examples, may be Hayem's solution or Gower's solution. Diluted blood is not stable and tests should be done within 2 hr of blood dilution (see Fig. 1.28).

For a platelet count, count tests should be done within 30 min of dilution.

(A)

BLOOD   DILUTING FLUID

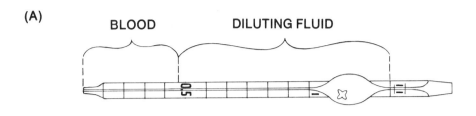

(B)

BLOOD   DILUTING FLUID

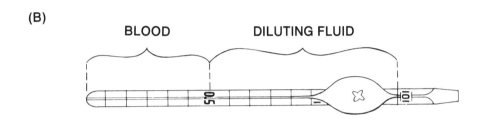

FIG. 1.28.   (A) WHITE CELL PIPETTE
(B) RED CELL PIPETTE

C. Blood Smear

Pick up 1 or 2 small drops of blood on one end of a slide. Place slide on a flat surface. Using a second slide as a spreader, make the blood smear. When the smear is dry, stain slide with Wright's stain to preserve the cells. The smear should be stained within 2 hr after it is made. The stain usually begins to fade after 2 years. The blood smear is used to examine the type, maturity and appearance of the white and red cells, respectively. The former is the differential white cell count and the latter the stained red cell examination. A platelet count can also be carried out on the blood smear. This will be more completely discussed in a later section.

D. Patient Care After Fingertip Puncture or Venipuncture

(See Section III, A.7, B.11 and B.14.)

VI. COAGULATION AND BLEEDING TIMES

Coagulation and bleeding time tests are nonspecific, since a deficiency in any of the factors involved in clot formation could vary the result.

A. Coagulation Time Tests on Capillary Blood

These tests are performed to check on abnormal clotting mechanism. The coagulation time is time required for blood to coagulate. The coagulation time will be performed by slide and capillary methods if using fingertip blood or Lee-White method if using venipuncture blood.

1.   Assemble Equipment for.—

a. Fingertip puncture as described previously
b. Coagulation tests—glass slides; several non-anticoagulated capillary tubes, 80 mm long × 1.0 mm in diameter; 2 stopwatches.

2.   Procedure.—

a. Puncture fingertip as described above and wipe away first drop of blood.

b. Slide Method.—
   (1)   Start one of the stopwatches and immediately collect 3 separate <u>large</u> drops of blood on a glass slide. Put slide aside for 2 min.
   (2)   After 2 min, and at 30 sec intervals thereafter, draw the lancet point through the drop of blood until you observe fibrin strands.
   (3)   When strands are noted, stop the stopwatch and record time and method on the hematology requisition slip. Normal coagulation time is 2–6 min by this method.

c. Capillary Method.—During the 2 min wait in the slide method, collect blood for the capillary method.

   (1)   Start the second stopwatch and fill by capillary action 2 capillary tubes 3/4 full of blood. Put one end of tube in the blood, the other end tilt down. Make a note of which capillary tube you filled first and which end you filled first.

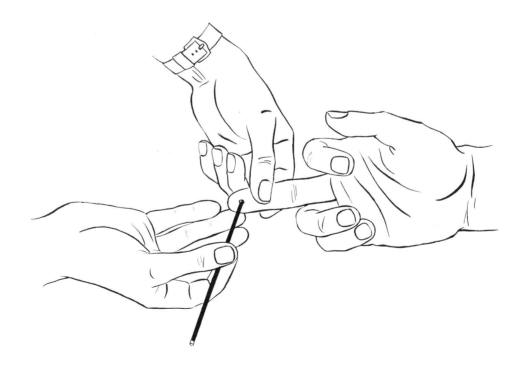

FIG. 1.29. FILLING A CAPILLARY TUBE

(2) Place capillary tubes on table undisturbed for 2 min.

(3) After 2 min, and at 30 sec intervals thereafter, carefully break the capillary tubes with both hands. Start on the capillary tube filled first and at end filled first. Try not to pull broken ends too far apart. Look for the thin fibrin strands between the broken ends.

(A) (B)

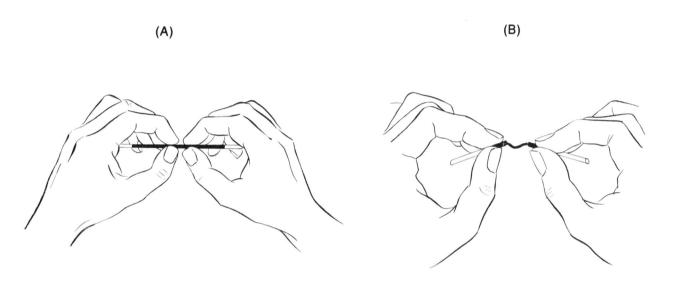

FIG. 1.30.   (A) BREAKING A CAPILLARY TUBE
(B) FIBRIN THREAD BETWEEN BROKEN ENDS OF CAPILLARY TUBE

(4) When fibrin is first seen, stop the stopwatch, record the time and method. Normal coagulation time is 2–6 min by this method.

   This method may fail to show a normal coagulation time if tissue juices mix with the blood on squeezing the fingertip. (*NOTE:* Student should complete the slide coagulation time during the 2 min wait for the capillary coagulation time.)

(5) *List of Precautions To Be Taken To Ensure Accuracy of the Capillary Coagulation Time Test.—*

   (a) Use non-heparinized or non-anticoagulated capillary tubes, otherwise blood will not coagulate.

(b)   Set stopwatch just as you put one end of capillary tube into the drop of blood.

(c)   Wait correct amount of time before breaking the capillary tube (2 min).

(d)   Break end of capillary tube that was filled first.

(e)   Do not pull broken ends of capillary tube too far apart, otherwise you will break the fibrin strands.

(f)   Fill up 2 capillary tubes, since blood might not coagulate by the time you completely break the first capillary tube.

(g)   Place capillary tubes on table without touching anything, otherwise blood may drain out of the capillary tube by capillary attraction.

(h)   Have extra capillary tubes available in case one breaks as you are filling it.

(i)   Hold capillary tube at a downward slant to facilitate filling of the tube.

(j)   Fill capillary tube only 2/3–3/4 full.

(k)   Record time accurately in minutes and seconds.

B.   Duke's Method for Bleeding Time on Capillary Blood

Duke's method is an example of a bleeding time test. The bleeding time is the time required for a small cut to stop bleeding. This test is dependent upon the functional ability of the platelets and capillary vasoconstriction to stop the bleeding. It is used before surgery to check for prolonged bleeding of the patient. The methods for testing bleeding time are crude and obsolete.

1.   Assemble Equipment for.—

a.   Fingertip puncture as described above

b.   Duke's method.—Piece of filter paper, stopwatch

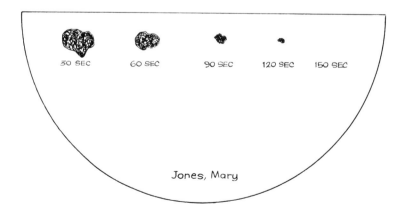

FIG. 1.31.   FILTER PAPER SHOWING THE RESULTS OF A NORMAL BLEEDING TIME BY DUKE'S METHOD

2. **Procedure.—**

a. Puncture fingertip as described previously; wipe away first drop of blood and allow blood to flow freely. Do not squeeze or massage the finger.

b. Start the stopwatch and at 30 sec intervals touch the filter paper to the blood coming out of the puncture. Do not touch the skin with the filter paper. As the bleeding ceases, the blood spot on the filter paper becomes smaller and smaller until bleeding stops, at which time no spot will be seen.

c. When bleeding stops, stop the stopwatch and record the time and method. Normal bleeding time is 1–3 min by this method.

Working in pairs, Student A punctures Student B, takes blood and performs slide and capillary coagulation times. Student B then punctures Student A, takes blood and performs capillary coagulation time and Duke's bleeding time.

C. Venipuncture Blood Coagulation Time—Lee-White Method

1. Assemble Equipment for.—

a. Venipuncture as described previously

b. Lee-White method.—Sterile physiological saline solution; 3 clean 8 mm diameter tubes, labeled 1, 2 and 3; test tube rack; 37°C water bath, stopwatch.

2. Procedure.—

a. Thoroughly rinse needle and syringe with sterile physiological saline solution. This allows space in needle and tip of syringe to be filled with saline and not air, since air hastens coagulation.

b. Perform a venipuncture as described previously. Attempt to enter the vein cleanly on the first attempt, since mixture of tissue juice hastens coagulation.

c. Withdraw blood slowly so no air bubbles pass through the blood.

d. Start the stopwatch as soon as blood is seen in the syringe.

e. Withdraw 5 ml of blood.

f. Remove needle from syringe.

g. Gently transfer 1 ml of blood to each of the 3 labeled test tubes. Blood should flow gently down wall of tube as excessive agitation will hasten coagulation.

h. Place the 3 test tubes in a 37°C water bath for 4 min.

i. When 4 min have elapsed, gently tilt tube 1 through an angle of 90°, at 30 sec intervals, until a clot is formed and blood will not flow from tube 1.

j. Tubes 2 and 3 are left undisturbed until coagulation occurs in the first tube. Then the second and third tubes are tilted in turn until coagulation has occurred.

k. When clot is formed in tube 3 and blood will not flow from tube 3, stop the stopwatch and record the time and method. The time is counted from time the blood enters the syringe until blood in tube 3 has coagulated. Three test tubes are used as each tube is subjected to less tilting and thus less agitation of the blood and so a more accurate coagulation time is achieved. Normal coagulation time for this method is 6–10 min.

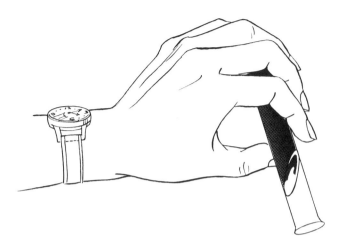

FIG. 1.32.   ENDPOINT OF LEE-WHITE COAGULATION TIME

3.   Possible Errors in Lee-White Method.—

a.   Coagulation Time Decreased Due To.—

(1) *Air Bubbles in the Blood.*—Caused by poor venipuncture. Needle loosely attached to syringe or needle not completely in the vein.

(2) *Tissue Juices Mixed with Blood.*—Caused by repeated punctures before penetrating the vein.

(3) *Dirty Test Tubes.*—Tube must be exceptionally clean and well rinsed with distilled water.

(4) *Excessive Agitation of the Blood.*—Occurs during transfer of blood from syringe to test tube. Blood should flow gently down inside of tube, not squirt into tube.

b.   Temperature Effect.—Coagulation time increased if temperature is below 35°C or above 45°C. Blood clots twice as fast at 37°C than at room temperature (25°C).

c.   Diameter of Test Tube.—Test tubes used must be of equal diameter as blood clots faster in smaller diameter tubes. Increased surface area of the glass (a foreign substance) to blood decreases coagulation time.

VII.   AUTOMATED PROCEDURES FOR THE COMPLETE BLOOD COUNT

The potential exists for performing any of the tests of the complete blood count, plus hematocrit and red cell indexes by use of automated equipment, such as the Coulter Counter (Model F or S), SMA counter (Hemalog), and Fisher Autocytometer. Several of these automated methods will be detailed in later exercises.

PROGRAMMED QUESTIONS

Cover answers with a piece of paper.   Answers appear at end of questions.

(1) The <u>basic</u> complete blood count consists of _____.
   (a) Hb, WBC, platelet count, differential
   (b) Stained red cell examination, reticulocyte count, Hb
   (c) WBC, differential, Hb, RBC
   (d) Differential, RBC, reticulocyte count, coagulation time

(2) Choose from the list below an incorrect step in the collecting of blood samples.
   (a) Assemble apparatus before collection
   (b) Clean the area from which collection is to be made with water
   (c) Be kind to the patient
   (d) Compare patient's hematology request form with patient's identification wrist band

(3) Why is a disposable sterile blood lancet used only once?
   (a) Prevent spread of hepatitis
   (b) Point becomes dull after use
   (c) It is no longer disposable if used more than once
   (d) None of the above

(4) During a venipuncture, when should the tourniquet be released?
   (a) After withdrawal of the needle
   (b) Before withdrawal of the needle
   (c) Before blood is transferred to test tube
   (d) While needle is being inserted into the vein

(5) Which of the following anticoagulants does <u>not</u> bind to Ca ions to prevent coagulation?
   (a) EDTA
   (b) Heparin
   (c) Sodium citrate
   (d) Oxalate

(6) In the Lee-White coagulation time method, which would retard coagulation?
   (a) Dirty test tubes
   (b) Temperature above 45°C
   (c) Tissue juices
   (d) Air bubble in blood

(7) What is the normal range of time for Duke's bleeding time method?
   (a) 2–6 min
   (b) 60–90 sec
   (c) 2–15 min
   (d) 1–3 min

(8) What does the alcohol swab at the end of a fingertip puncture procedure for collection of blood accomplish?
   (a) Alcohol stops bleeding of the wound immediately
   (b) Alcohol disinfects wound
   (c) Alcohol allows Ca ions to become bound
   (d) None of above, as alcohol does not disinfect the wound

(9) In preparing the vacutainer for venipuncture, where should the top of rubber stopper of the vacutainer be set before the needle is inserted into the vein?
  (a) At the guide line on the vacutainer holder
  (b) Depressed to end of the vacutainer holder
  (c) At the middle of the vacutainer holder
  (d) At the beginning of the vacutainer holder

(10) Which vein of the forearm is most frequently used for venipuncture?
  (a) Femoral
  (b) Superior vena cava
  (c) Median cubital
  (d) Carotid

Answers

(1) c
(2) b
(3) a
(4) b
(5) b

(6) b
(7) d
(8) b
(9) a
(10) c

Hemoglobinometry

Hemoglobin is a pigment within the red cell primarily involved in carrying oxygen.

I. NORMAL HEMOGLOBIN VALUES

The hemoglobin value is often proportional to the red cell count. The concentration of hemoglobin in adults varies somewhat with the sex of the individual.

Males	14–16 g/100 ml blood
Females	11–14 g/100 ml blood
Children	11–12 g/100 ml blood
Infants	14–20 g/100 ml blood

The average value for adults is 14.5 g Hb/100 ml blood.

II. GENERAL PRINCIPLES OF HEMOGLOBIN ESTIMATION

In most procedures used to estimate hemoglobin concentration a measured volume of blood is pipetted into a given volume of diluting solution. The diluting solution functions to:

(1) Break up or hemolyze the red cells
(2) Liberate hemoglobin
(3) Stabilize hemoglobin from decomposition by converting the hemoglobin to some other form.

In older procedures the last function was not considered, which led to erroneous results.

The stabilized hemoglobin molecule colors the diluting solution. The depth of color is proportional to the concentration of the hemoglobin molecules. The measurement is performed in an instrument known as a colorimeter by comparing the unknown sample of hemoglobin to a standard or known amount of hemoglobin.

III. METHODS OF HEMOGLOBIN ESTIMATION

There are two groups of colorimetric methods to estimate hemoglobin concentration.

A. Visual Colorimetric Methods

The visual colorimetric methods are relatively inaccurate and mainly of historical interest only. These will be listed but not discussed here.

1. **Direct-reading Tallqvist Method**
2. **Spencer Method**
3. **Haden-Hausser Method**

4. **Sahli-Hellige or Sahli Method.**—This method will be discussed as it is still used by some physicians and as an emergency technique.

   a. **Theory and Chemistry.**—The test is inaccurate because of errors in performance and the presence of nonhemoglobin substances in the blood which influence the color of the blood. The instrument used is the Sahli hemometer. In this method 0.1N HCl is the diluting fluid. The HCl hemolyzes the red cells and frees the hemoglobin. The released hemoglobin is stabilized by the HCl by conversion of hemoglobin to acid hematin, a stable form of hemoglobin which is tan in color.

$$\text{hemoglobin (red)} \xrightarrow{\quad \text{HCl} \quad} \text{acid hematin (tan)}$$

   The color obtained in the sample is matched against a color standard, consisting of two prisms of permanent tan-colored glass. One can easily convert from grams Hb to percent or vice versa by the following equation

$$\frac{14.5\,g}{100\%} = \frac{x\,(g)}{x\,(\%)}$$

   or by referring to the conversion table (Table 2.1). If a Sahli tube is used and is calibrated other than 14.5 g = 100%, the same equation applies by using substitution.

TABLE 2.1

THE SAHLI-HELLIGE CONVERSION TABLE

Grams	10	10.5	11	11.5	12	12.5	13	13.5	14
% of Normal	69.0	72.4	75.7	79.3	82.8	86.2	89.7	93.1	96.6

Grams	14.5	15	15.5	16	16.5	17	17.5	18	18.5
% of Normal	100.0	103.5	106.9	110.4	113.8	117.2	120.7	124.1	127.6

b. Method.—

(1) 0.1N HCl is placed in the Sahli tube to the 4 g mark, so match point (described later) is not passed when making comparison of unknown to standard (see below).

(2) Using a clean, dry Sahli or hemoglobin pipette, pipette <u>exactly</u> 20 mm^3 or 0.020 ml of blood from a fingertip puncture or from a tube of anticoagulated blood.

(3) Expel this blood directly into the diluting fluid with no bubbles. Rinse pipette 3 or 4 times with diluting fluid from the Sahli tube to remove all blood from the pipette. Keep tip of pipette under the surface of the diluting fluid while expelling the blood and rinsing the pipette.

(4) Set the timer for 5 min.

(5) Mix contents by swirling. If clots are present red cells will not be hemolyzed and the hemoglobin freed. A clotted sample can not be read.

(6) After 5 min have elapsed, add distilled water 1 or 2 drops at a time. Mix thoroughly after each addition with stirring rod or by gentle shaking until color of solution matches color of glass standard while holding the Sahli instrument up to a constant fluorescent light source to compare unknown to standard. When the match point between unknown and standard has been obtained, take the reading corresponding to height to which solution has risen in the Sahli tube. One side of the Sahli tube is calibrated in g Hb/100 ml blood. The other side of the Sahli tube is calibrated in percent hemoglobin with 14.5 g equivalent to 100% hemoglobin. (*NOTE:* Other Sahli tubes are calibrated differently. The 14.5 g = 100% is most frequently used.)

(7) Report the method and concentration of hemoglobin as g/100 ml blood and, if desired, as percent hemoglobin.

c. Disadvantages of Sahli Method.—

(1) Gradual addition of drops of water is time-consuming.

(2) If match point is passed, test has to be repeated.

(3) Test is inaccurate because of difficulty in making color comparisons between sample and standard due to amount of light coming through the back of the instrument. It is important to standardize the light source by holding the colorimeter at arm's length to a fluorescent light of constant intensity.

(4) Difficulty in matching sample to standard due to personal visual competency of the technician.

d. List of Precautions To Be Taken To Ensure Accuracy of Sahli Hemoglobin Estimation.—

(1) Constant light source

(2) Proper concentration of acid (0.1N HCl)

(3) Add distilled water 1 drop at a time so it does not pass the match point; stir after each drop.

(4) Specific timing of test (5 min)

B. Photoelectric Colorimetric Methods

These are the methods of choice today. These methods involve the use of an electronic colorimeter, either a spectrophotometer or a photometer. If these instruments are operating properly and standards are accurate, the results are highly reliable and preferred to other methods.

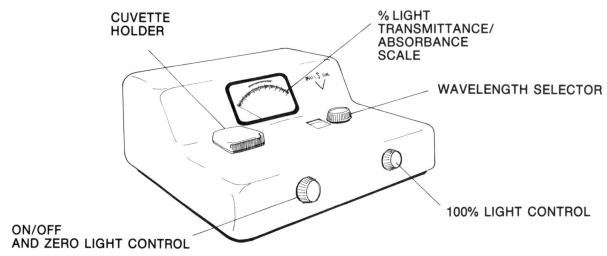

FIG. 2.1. BAUSCH AND LOMB SPECTRONIC "20"

1.   Principles of Spectrophotometry.—

a. A wavelength selector or diffraction grating filters out all but one wavelength of light from a white light source. This is known as a wavelength of monochromatic light.

b. This wavelength of monochromatic light passes through the solution containing the colored molecules, whose concentration you want to estimate. Some of the light is absorbed by the molecules of the solution and some of the light is transmitted.

c. The transmitted light strikes a photoelectric cell, which converts light energy to electrical energy. The photoelectric cell sends out an electric current which is proportional to the intensity of the transmitted light. The amount of electric current produced is measured and read out on a galvanometer whose scale is calibrated to read percentage of light transmitted.

The more concentrated (darker) the sample in solution, the more light is absorbed, and the less is the percentage of transmitted light. The less concentrated (lighter) the sample in solution, the less light is absorbed, and the greater is the percentage of transmitted light.

The colorimetric tests are valid only if color development is directly proportional to concentration of the substance in solution. Furthermore, time for color development must be exactly controlled, since color development continues with time. You must "read" the results in the spectrophotometer after a specified time.

In summary, the intensity of a beam of monochromatic light entering and leaving a solution depends on the concentration of the light-absorbing molecules in the solution. This is known as Beer's Law or the Beer-Lambert Law. For a more complete discussion of photometry see series *Laboratory Manual of Clinical Chemistry*.

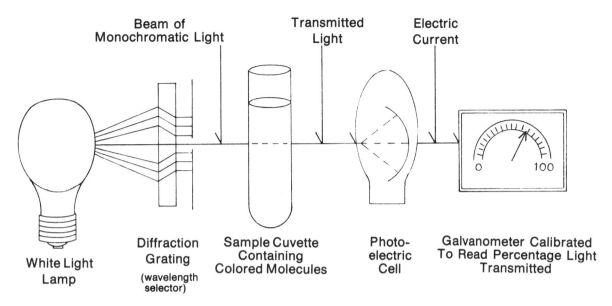

FIG. 2.2. SCHEMATIC OF A SPECTROPHOTOMETER

2. **Standard or Calibration Curve.**—The spectrophotometer must be checked out before using to determine if it is operating properly. This is accomplished through preparation of a standard or calibration curve. A standard curve is only good for that one specific instrument for that day.

To prepare a standard curve, begin with an accurate stock standard solution of known concentration of the substance you want to measure. From the stock solution, prepare 3 or 4 accurate dilutions of different known concentrations; these are the diluted standards. Begin with the lowest concentration, proceed to the highest concentration and read the percentage of light transmitted for each of the standards. The percent light transmission is then plotted against concentration of the substance on semilog graph paper. If concentration of the substance is directly proportional to depth of color, then a line drawn through the points for the standards should be a straight line and should pass through 100% light transmission, which is zero concentration for the molecules of the substance.

Example: Preparation of Standard Curve for Hemoglobin Estimation. Using the Bausch and Lomb (B and L) Spectronic 20 as the spectrophotometer and Hycel cyanmethemoglobin as the standard, the standard curve is prepared. The cyanmethemoglobin method of Drabkin is commonly considered to be the most accurate method in use today.

Dilutions of Hycel cyanmethemoglobin stock standard are made with Hycel cyanmethemoglobin reagent to prepare the diluted standard solutions. Make dilution in labeled cuvette as follows.

Blood (g Hb/100 ml)	Volume of Stock Standard (ml)	Volume of Reagent (ml)
0 (blank)	0	6.0
5	1.5	4.5
10	3.0	3.0
15	4.5	1.5
20	6.0	0

Read the percent light transmission (%T) for each standard from lowest to highest and plot %T versus g Hb/100 ml blood on semilog graph paper. To read the standards, see methods following in Section 3b.

Standards (g Hb/100 ml Blood)	%T
5	71
10	51
15	36
20	25

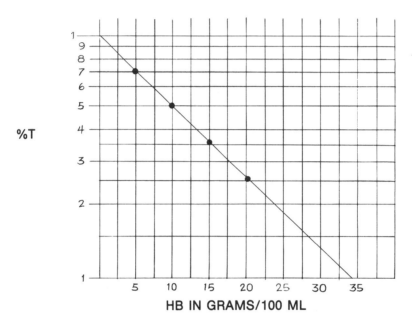

FIG. 2.3. STANDARD CURVE FOR HEMOGLOBIN BY CYANMETHEMOGLOBIN METHOD

In addition to making sure the instrument is reliable, the standard curve is used to read the unknown sample values (in g Hb/100 ml blood) after the percent light transmission is recorded from the spectrophotometer.

3. Cyanmethemoglobin Method for Hemoglobin Estimation (Drabkin's Method).—

a. **Principles (Chemistry) of Drabkin's Method.**—The diluting fluid is Drabkin's solution. It consists of sodium bicarbonate ($NaHCO_3$) 1.0 g, potassium cyanide (KCN) 0.05 g, potassium ferricyanide ($K_3Fe(CN)_6$) 0.20 g, and distilled water 1000 ml. (This solution is available commercially in liquid form or dry pack.)

NOTE: A word of caution about Drabkin's solution—Drabkin's solution contains cyanide. It must be pipetted either with a rubber bulb attached to the pipette or by an autodiluter or from a burette, but NEVER BY MOUTH.

Drabkin's solution is only good for 3 weeks to 1 month, since ferricyanide breaks down and cyanide, being a gas, evaporates into the air. Store Drabkin's solution in a cool place and in a brown bottle to exclude light.

When a volume of blood is placed in Drabkin's solution, the blood cells are hemolyzed and the hemoglobin is freed. The ferricyanide in the Drabkin's solution stabilizes the hemoglobin by converting the hemoglobin's iron from the ferrous state (Fe^{++}) to the ferric state (Fe^{+++}) to form the methemoglobin compound.

$$Hb\,(Fe^{++}) \xrightarrow{\text{ferricyanide}} Hb\,(Fe^{+++})$$
$$\text{hemoglobin} \qquad\qquad\qquad \text{methemoglobin}$$

The cyanide in the Drabkin's solution then converts the methemoglobin to cyanmethemoglobin.

$$Hb\,(Fe^{+++}) \xrightarrow{\text{KCN}} Hb\,(Fe^{+++})\,CN$$
$$\text{methemoglobin} \qquad\qquad \text{cyanmethemoglobin}$$

The depth of color of the cyanmethemoglobin solution is proportional to the concentration of the cyanmethemoglobin and to the hemoglobin from which it was formed. Thus, we can measure the concentration of hemoglobin in the solution by the spectrophotometer.

b. Method.—

(1) Before beginning the estimation of hemoglobin, the spectrophotometer (B and L Spectronic 20 or other spectrophotometer) is turned on and warmed up 10–15 min. The wavelength selector is set to 540 millimicrons (mμ) or nanometers (nm). This monochromatic wavelength of light is greenish-yellow in color.

(2) The solutions for hemoglobin estimation are placed in matched cuvettes. Matched cuvettes allow the same amount of light to pass through since their walls are of the same composition of glass, uniformly of same thickness, not scratched, clean and dry.

(3) The spectrophotometer is "zeroed" into 0 without a cuvette in the cuvette holder with the lid closed and then "set" to 100% light transmission with a "blank" cuvette in the cuvette holder. A "blank" cuvette contains Drabkin's solution plus a volume of distilled water in the same amount as blood is added in a sample determination. This is done so that the total volume of "blank" and samples are the same.

(4) After the spectrophotometer has been adjusted, the standards are read (they have been previously prepared as described in Fig. 2.3 standard curve above) and the standard curve is prepared (%T versus g Hb/100 ml blood). Then the hemoglobin estimation of the unknown blood samples can be carried out.

(5) Into matched cuvettes, pipette with the autodiluter 5 ml of Drabkin's solution for the blank and each unknown sample. Place cuvettes into a rubberized test tube rack (Kahn racks) to prevent scratching the tubes.

(6) To one Drabkin's filled cuvette, add exactly 20 mm³ (0.02 ml) of distilled water. This tube serves as the "blank."

	Blank		Sample Determination
Drabkin's solution	5 ml		Drabkin's solution
Distilled water	20 mm^3		Blood

(7) Add to the other cuvettes exactly 20 mm^3 of blood from a fingertip puncture or from a tube of anticoagulated blood by using a clean and dry Sahli or hemoglobin pipette.

(8) Expel this blood immediately into the Drabkin's solution. Rinse pipette 3–4 times with Drabkin's solution from the cuvette to remove all the blood from the pipette. Keep tip of pipette under the surface of the diluting solution while expelling the blood and rinsing the pipette.

(9) Set the timer for 10 min.

(10) Mix the contents by vigorous swirling. Cuvette is left standing for 10 min to permit formation of cyanmethemoglobin.

(11) After 10 min have elapsed, zero spectrophotometer to 0 with zero adjust-control knob. Place "blank" cuvette into cuvette holder with line-up mark facing raised ridge on cuvette holder. Close the lid; with light control knob set the instrument to read 100% light transmission.

(12) The samples are then placed in the spectrophotometer and the percent light transmissions are read off for each one. The unknown sample percent light transmissions are referred to the standard curve to obtain their concentrations in g Hb/100 ml blood.

The more concentrated the hemoglobin in solution, the more light is absorbed; the less light passes through the solution, the lower the percent light transmission reading on the galvanometer will be. The less concentrated the hemoglobin in solution, the less light is absorbed; the more light passes through the solution, the higher the percent light transmission reading on the galvanometer will be.

c. **Errors in Hemoglobinometry.**—Errors can occur in:

(1) Sample
(2) Method
(3) Equipment—not using matched cuvettes
(4) Errors of technician

d. **List of Precautions To Be Taken To Ensure Accuracy of Drabkin's Hemoglobin Estimation.**—(Some of these precautions also apply to the Sahli method.)

(1) Accurate pipetting (20 mm^3); wipe outside of pipette; tease blood to mark. Allow no air bubbles in the pipette.
(2) Use clean, dry, unbroken pipettes.
(3) Place pipette below surface of diluting fluid on expelling the blood, so all blood is hemolyzed.

(4) Exact timing of the test (10 min).

(5) Rinse pipette with diluting fluid several times to clear pipette of all traces of blood.

(6) Swirl tube vigorously to prevent clotting of the blood.

(7) Warm up spectrophotometer for 5–10 min before using.

(8) Set wavelength at 540 millimicrons (mμ) or nanometers (nm).

(9) Use matched cuvettes.

(10) Use fresh Drabkin's solution—not over 1 month old.

(11) Use correct volume of Drabkin's solution (5 ml).

(12) Standardize or calibrate spectrophotometer correctly by using fresh standards.

(13) Have spectrophotometer "zeroed in" properly, first without and then set to 100% T with the blank.

(14) Read and record results accurately.

e. Clinical Significance Versus Performance Accuracy.—For example, if average value for a test is 5 and your reading for a particular patient is 8, is this value clinically significant? The value might be clinically significant if the value for the patient falls outside of the limits established by the standard deviation from the mean, which for medical and biological studies is usually the $M \pm 2$ S.D.

If, on the other hand, the average value for a test is 5 and your reading for this patient is 4.5, this is considered performance accuracy and is not clinically significant. This tells us the closeness with which this particular result agrees with the value accepted as true for this specific test.

f. Quality Control.—Quality control is an absolute necessity in the hematology laboratory with the introduction of electronic automated equipment. The objectives of a quality control program are to keep a surveillance on the accuracy and precision of test procedures.

In considering errors in a specific test procedure and in establishing quality control programs, the terms accuracy and precision, which are not synonymous, and standards and reference controls are frequently used.

(1) Accuracy.—Accuracy means the closeness with which the test procedure is able to approach the true or correct value of a standard. A standard is a substance of known composition, the value of which was estimated by a test procedure different from that usually used in the clinical laboratory. The standard checks on the reliability of a test procedure. The standards are obtained from sources outside of the laboratory. Accuracy implies freedom from error.

(2) Precision.—Precision means the closeness with which a test procedure is able to duplicate the same result on repeated analysis on samples of a reference control. A reference control resembles the unknown specimen but contains various substances of known concentrations, the values of which are estimated by the test procedure usually used in the clinical laboratory. The reference controls are variable in their composition and are not constant as standards. The reference controls are tested together with the unknown samples and

they check on the reproducibility of a test procedure. The results on the reference control form the basis for the calculation of the mean and standard deviation of a given test procedure.

As an example in comparing precision to accuracy, if it is possible to perform consecutive tests on a substance with excellent reproducibility, this is precision. However, if the instrument on which the analyses were performed was incorrectly calibrated there would be a constant error in the values and thus a lack of accuracy or reliability. The standard should be used to check on accuracy of the instrument.

Precision of a specific test procedure can be estimated by calculating the mean and standard deviations and then plotting a quality control or range chart. The standard deviation describes the spread of individual values of the reference control compared to the average. The greater the difference between the individual determinations and the average value, the less the precision of the method. For medical and biological studies a test procedure is in control, i.e., the test procedure has precision, if the values for the reference control fall within the $M \pm 2$ S.D. When values fall outside these limits, the test procedure is considered out of control.

The reference control for hemoglobin is a stable solution of hemolyzed red cells, such as Globintrol. This solution is carried through all the steps of the procedure just as for any unknown sample and should pick up errors within the specific test procedure (e.g., cyanmethemoglobin). The values for the Globintrol should fall within ± 2 S.D. of the mean (M) assay value given on the package. The Globintrol should be done in duplicate determinations daily, treated exactly the same as unknown specimens and given no preferential treatment. After several results are obtained, the mean and the standard deviations can be calculated and plotted on a quality control chart (see Fig. 2.4).

Note from the chart that during days 1–6, the values are well within normal control limits as they cluster around the mean. Days 7–10 values are in normal range but fluctuate considerably, which might indicate that somewhere in the procedure some factor might be fluctuating, such as in the spectrophotometer.

On days 11–21, values have a definite upward trend, which might be due to deterioration of reagents. At arrow on day 22, new reagents were made up, and on days 23–26, good control is obtained again. On day 27 a value was obtained outside control limits and this would require immediate attention to find the cause and repeat the analysis of controls and unknowns.

By instituting a quality control program, degree of precision of a test procedure and the ability to measure accuracy of a test procedure can be checked. By plotting a quality control chart, inaccuracies, trends, intermittent problems, and test bias can be detected and corrective steps taken.

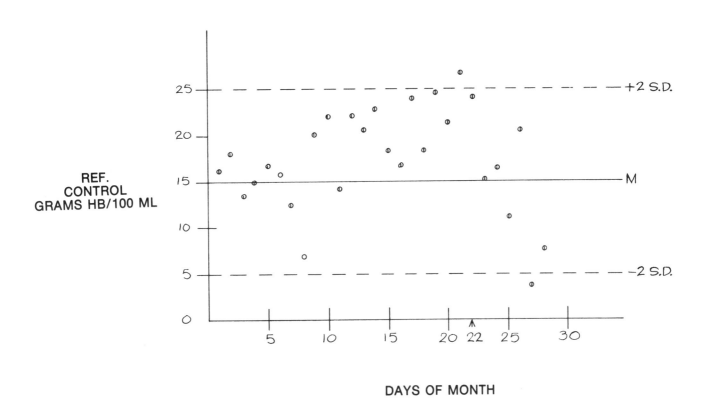

FIG. 2.4.   QUALITY CONTROL CHARTS FOR GLOBINTROL BY CYANMETHEMOGLOBIN METHOD

PROGRAMMED QUESTIONS

Cover answers with a piece of paper.   Answers appear at end of questions.

(1) What is <u>one</u> function of the diluting solution in <u>any</u> hemoglobin method?
  (a) Preserve the red cells
  (b) Hemolyze the red cells
  (c) Maintain the hemoglobin intact
  (d) Precipitate the hemoglobin

(2) In the Sahli-Hellige method hemoglobin
is converted to _____.
  (a) Cyanmethemoglobin
  (b) Alkaline hematin
  (c) Sulfhematin
  (d) Acid hematin

(3) Choose from the list below one function of the standard curve.
(a) To read off unknown sample values after %T is recorded
(b) To determine reliability of the standards
(c) To convert g Hb/100 ml blood to %T
(d) None of the above

(4) What wavelength is used in the cyanmethemoglobin method?
(a) 620 mμ
(b) 450 mμ
(c) 540 mμ
(d) 360 mμ

(5) Drabkin's solution contains _____.
(a) Copper sulfate
(b) Cyanide
(c) Hydrochloric acid
(d) Potassium bicarbonate

(6) What volume of blood is used in the method of Drabkin or Sahli?
(a) 20 mm^3
(b) 0.5 ml
(c) 5 ml
(d) 10 ml

(7) Which component of the spectrophotometer allows for a wavelength of monochromatic light?
(a) Photoelectric cell
(b) Cuvette
(c) Colored glass standard
(d) Diffraction grating (monochromator)

(8) When iron is in the Fe^{+++} state the molecule is called?
(a) Hemoglobin
(b) Methemoglobin
(c) Reduced hemoglobin
(d) Oxyhemoglobin

(9) What is the function of a "blank" cuvette in the spectrophotometer?
(a) To "set" the instrument to read 0% T on the galvanometer
(b) To "set" the photoelectric cell to give off maximum white light
(c) To "set" the instrument to read 100% T on the galvanometer
(d) To "set" the colored glass standards to read 100% T on the galvanometer

(10) What does the term precision in quality control mean?
(a) Reproducibility
(b) Standardization
(c) Reliability
(d) Freedom from error

Answers

(1) b	(6) a
(2) d	(7) d
(3) a	(8) b
(4) c	(9) c
(5) b	(10) a

Differential White Blood Cell Count

The value of the differential white cell count depends on the proper preparation and staining of the blood smear.

I. PREPARATION OF THE BLOOD SMEAR

A. Procedure

1. **Slide Method.—**

   a. Glass slides must be perfectly clean, dry and grease-free. Handle slides only by their edges.

   b. Make 2 blood smears (1 is held in reserve in case original is broken or double check is desired).

   c. A fingertip puncture is made, the first drop of blood wiped away. Work quickly to avoid clotting.

   d. Pick up 1 or 2 <u>small</u> drops of blood about 1/2 in. from one end of the slide.

   e. Place slide on a flat surface with drop of blood at your right (for right-handed people).

   f. Place the second "spreader" slide in the middle of the first slide. Hold "spreader" slide at a 25° angle and draw the spreader slide toward the drop(s) of blood to contact the blood. (*NOTE:* Some more expensive slide boxes include a special slide spreader with beveled edge. Automatic blood spreaders are now available.)

   g. Allow the blood to spread out under edge of the spreader slide by capillary attraction. Then with an <u>even, rapid, smooth</u> movement <u>push</u> the "spreader" slide to the left along the first <u>slide</u>. The blood will follow and form a thin, uniform smear.

   h. Allow smear to air dry. Drying may be hastened by waving slide in the air. The quicker the drying, the less the distortion of the cells.

   i. Label thick end of smear with patient's name <u>in pencil</u>. The thick end of the smear is the end from which the smear was made. The thin end or "feathered" end of the smear is opposite.

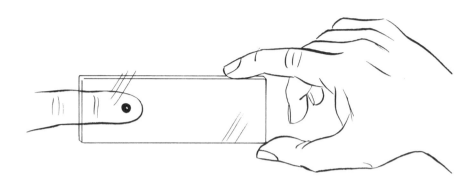

FIG. 3.1.   METHOD OF PICKING UP DROPS OF BLOOD

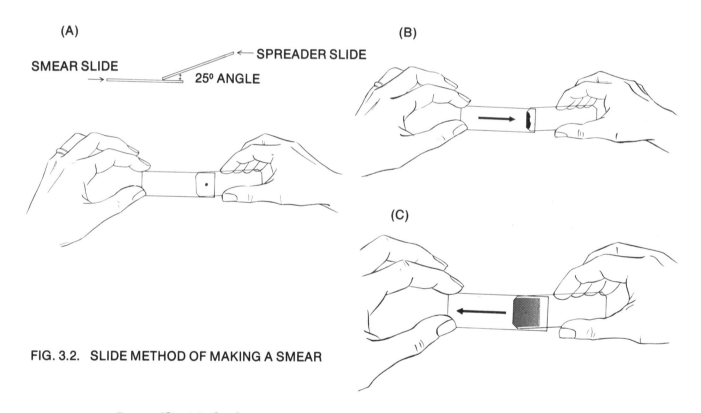

(A)

SMEAR SLIDE
← SPREADER SLIDE
25° ANGLE

(B)

(C)

FIG. 3.2.   SLIDE METHOD OF MAKING A SMEAR

2.   **Cover Slip Method.—**

   a.   Hold 2 cover slips by their edges with thumb and forefinger of each hand.
   b.   Touch the center of the cover slip to a small drop of blood.
   c.   Immediately the second cover slip is diagonally superimposed.
   d.   The blood spreads by capillary attraction between the 2 cover slips. Just before the spreading has almost stopped, evenly and smoothly draw the cover slips apart in the horizontal plane (see Fig. 3.3).

e.   Place smears up to air dry and then stain. The cover slip method supposedly gives a better distribution of the leukocytes.

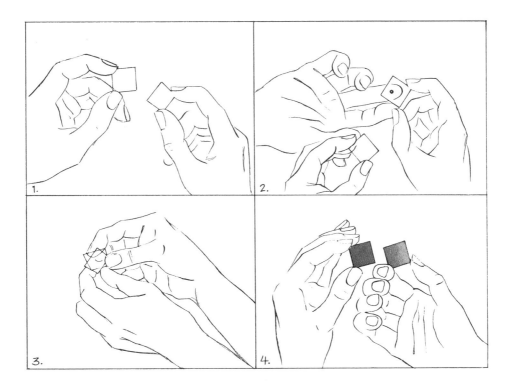

FIG. 3.3.   COVER SLIP METHOD OF MAKING A BLOOD SMEAR

B.   Criteria of a Good Blood Smear

1.   Thick area makes a gradual transition to thin area. Blood smear is a reasonable thickness and length. The smear should be smooth and without waves. Concentric crescent-shaped rings may be seen.
2.   The "feathered" end of the smear does not extend to end of the slide. There are margins at top and bottom of the smear.
3.   Smear is smooth in appearance.

C.   Causes of a Poor Blood Smear

1.   Drop of blood is too large.
2.   "Spreader" slide is pushed with a jerky motion.
3.   "Spreader" slide is not pushed rapidly enough. The spreader slide should be pushed with same speed as a match is struck.
4.   "Feathered" end extends to end of the slide.
5.   Smear dried too slowly; cells are distorted.
6.   Lack of smooth appearance of smear due to use of rough-edged spreader slide and greasy slide.

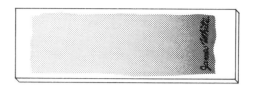

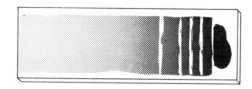

FIG. 3.4.   GOOD VERSUS POOR SMEAR

D. Factors That Determine Thinness of the Blood Smear

1. **Angle of Spreader Slide.**—The greater the angle, the thicker the smear.
2. **Pressure Placed on the "Spreader" Slide.**—The greater the pressure, the thinner the smear.
3. **Rapidity of Spreading Motion.**—The greater the rapidity, the thinner the smear.
4. **Size of Drop of Blood.**—The greater the size, the thicker the smear.

II. STAINING OF THE BLOOD SMEAR

A. Wright's Stain

The examination of the cells of the blood smear is facilitated by staining of the smear. In this way the various cells become easily differentiated. The common stain used is Wright's stain.

1. **Fixation.**—Wright's stain combines fixation of the cells, which preserves the cells, and staining of the cells. A good fixative for the blood smear is methyl alcohol. Since Wright's stain is dissolved in methyl alcohol, fixation takes place when the Wright's stain is first applied. The methyl alcohol should be anhydrous and acetone free.

2. **Stain.**—The Wright's stain and other stains to be discussed below are polychromatic stains, since they produce a variety of colors.
    a. The polychromatic nature of these stains is due to the methylene blue component of the stain, which gives rise to azure A, azure B and methylene violet. The polychromatic stain is a mixture of all these dyes and is responsible for the color range that is observed on staining. In Wright's stain the polychroming of the methylene

blue occurs by "aging" the stain at an alkaline pH or by heating the stain in alkaline solution. As a result of the "aging" process, the amounts of azure stains are unknown, and non-uniform staining from one day to another usually results.

b. If one wants to ensure more uniform staining results, solutions of known composition and weights of azures can be prepared, for example, Giemsa's stain. A stock solution of the stain is dissolved in a mixture of glycerol and absolute methyl alcohol. The stock stain is then diluted with phosphate buffer (pH 6.8) to permit ionization of the stains. The stains are alcoholic solutions of basic and acidic components.

(1) **Methylene Blue.**—A basic stain, which stains nuclei and some cytoplasmic structures blue. The blue-stained structures are basophilic substances.

(2) **Eosin.**—An acidic stain, which stains some cytoplasmic structures red. The red-staining structures are acidophilic or eosinophilic substances.

(3) When both the basic and the acidic stains stain the cytoplasmic structures, a pink to lilac color develops; these structures are neutrophilic substances.

(4) **Mode of Staining Action.**—The mode of action of the stain depends on dissociation of the stain components after mixing with the buffer. If buffer is too acidic, it allows the eosin to dissociate too much, thus to stain too brightly, and therefore the basic stain too faintly. If the buffer is too basic, it allows the methylene blue to dissociate too much, thus to stain too brightly, and therefore the acidic stain too faintly. In the staining process, the buffer solution must control the acid-base balance of the stain to give the proper coloration to the components of the blood cells.

B. Staining Procedures

1. Manual Procedure.—

a. Place slide on staining rack with smear side up. Be sure patient's identification is on slide.

b. Cover the blood smear with Wright's stain. Set timer for 3 min.

c. Then add 5 drops of Giordano's phosphate buffer (pH 6.4) for 5 min. (Some prefer to use ordinary tap water.) Do not wash off the Wright's stain. The times given may vary depending on the particular batch of stain.

d. Mix buffer and stain by gently blowing a stream of air on the slide during the first minute. If mixing is proper a greenish, mixed metallic sheen should appear on the surface. The stain-buffer mixture should not run off the slide.

e. After 5 min, add distilled water in a gentle stream to float off the metallic sheen.

f. Then flush with water more vigorously for 1 or 2 min.

g. Drain water from slide and allow to air dry. Do not blot surface of the smear as you will scratch the surface.

(A)

(B)

(C)

(D)

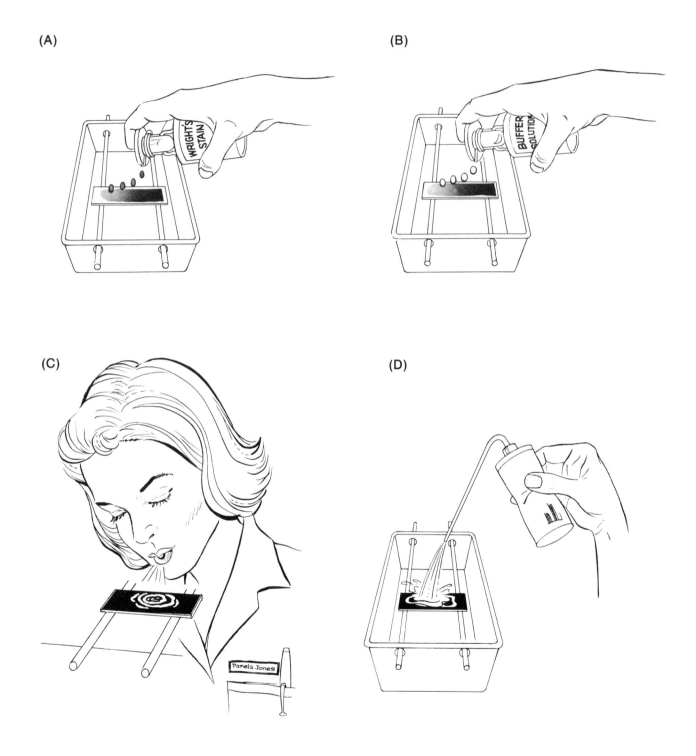

FIG. 3.5. METHOD FOR MANUAL STAINING
(A) Applying Wright's stain.   (C) Mixing stain and buffer.
(B) Adding buffer.   (D) Washing stain from slide.

2. **Automatic Procedure.**—There are many automatic staining procedures. Only the Hema-tek system is discussed here. After the instrument has been primed, the dried blood smears are placed in the slots at the loading point facing left, with "feathered" end away from you. When a smear advances into position face down on the staining plate, a switch activates the first pump, which delivers stain to the smear. The slide is stained by the stain's spreading between the metal plate and the surface of the smear. The smear advances to the second position and activates a second pump which delivers buffer. The stain and buffer mix as smear advances. It then starts a third pump, which delivers distilled water to rinse smear. The smear is dried by a current of warm air at the end of the plate, dropped off and stored in a collecting drawer. Twenty-five slides can be stained in about 30 min.

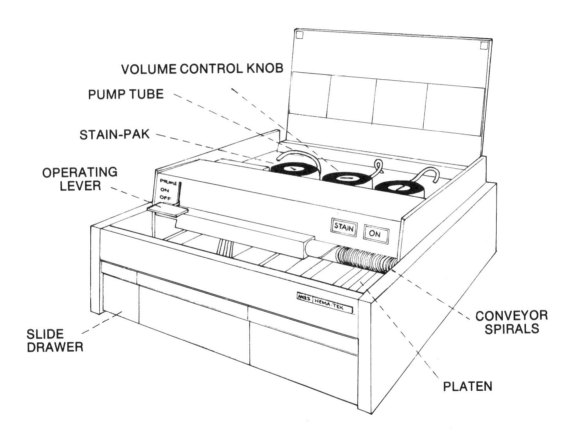

FIG. 3.6. HEMA-TEK SLIDE STAINER

C. Giemsa Stain, Polychrome Stain, Etc.

Since Wright's stain is the one most commonly used in the laboratory, other methods will not be described here. Any basic hematology reference book will describe other methods.

III. CELL IDENTIFICATION—CYTOLOGY OF CIRCULATING BLOOD CELLS

To the naked eye the blood smear after staining should appear pink or pinkish-violet. The thin end of the smear, where the cells are uniformly distributed, is examined under the oil immersion lens of the microscope. In cell identification keep four factors in mind: size of cell, features of the nucleus, features of the cytoplasmic granules, and nuclear/cytoplasmic ratio. In the descriptions that follow, colors of the constituents of the cells are based on staining with Wright's stain.

A. Erythrocyte —Mature Red Blood Cell

The cell is a nonnucleated, biconcave disk. Its cytoplasm is pink to red staining, light in the center with darker periphery.

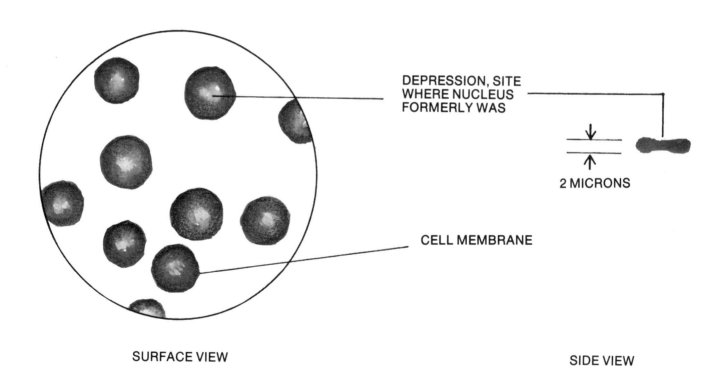

SURFACE VIEW   SIDE VIEW

FIG. 3.7. ERYTHROCYTES—MATURE RED CELLS (SEE COLOR ATLAS)

B. Leukocytes

Leukocytes are spherical shaped as suspended in the plasma, except for monocytes which are oval to irregular shaped (compare to Fig. 3.14). Leukocytes have a light blue staining cytoplasm, except for the neutrophil's cytoplasm, which is stained light pink.

1.   **Granulocytes.—**

   a.   **Neutrophils.—**

      (1)   Band cell or stab cell—immature neutrophil

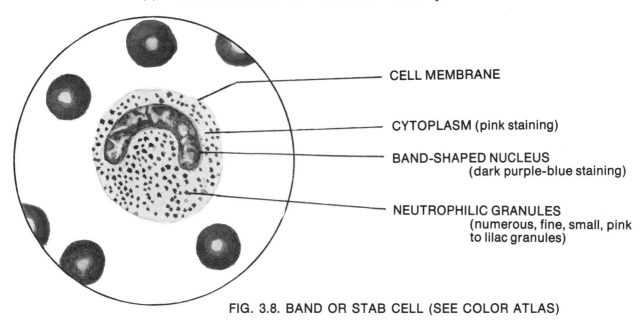

FIG. 3.8. BAND OR STAB CELL (SEE COLOR ATLAS)

      (2)   Mature neutrophil(e) (segmented neutrophil, polymorphonuclear leukocyte)

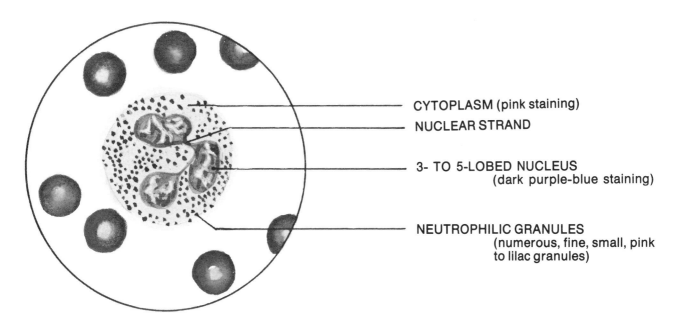

FIG. 3.9. MATURE NEUTROPHIL(E) OR POLYMORPHONUCLEAR LEUKOCYTE (SEE COLOR ATLAS)

   The mature neutrophil is also called segmented neutrophil because of the lobed condition of the nucleus. It is also termed polymorphonuclear leukocyte since the number of lobes of the nucleus varies with age of the cell.

b. Eosinophil(e)

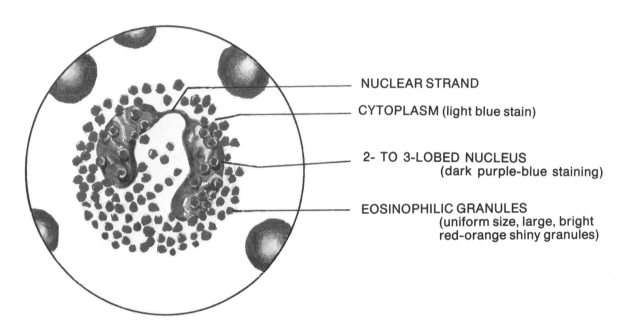

NUCLEAR STRAND

CYTOPLASM (light blue stain)

2- TO 3-LOBED NUCLEUS
(dark purple-blue staining)

EOSINOPHILIC GRANULES
(uniform size, large, bright
red-orange shiny granules)

FIG. 3.10. EOSINOPHIL(E) (SEE COLOR ATLAS)

c. Basophil(e)

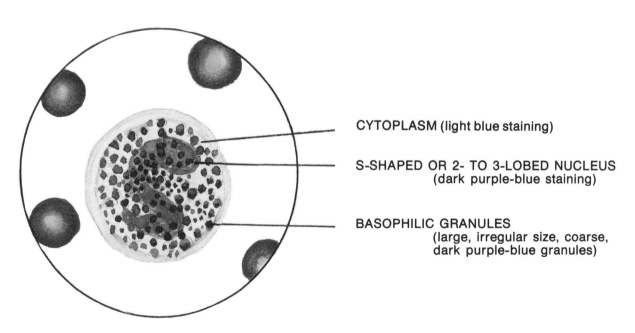

CYTOPLASM (light blue staining)

S-SHAPED OR 2- TO 3-LOBED NUCLEUS
(dark purple-blue staining)

BASOPHILIC GRANULES
(large, irregular size, coarse,
dark purple-blue granules)

FIG. 3.11. BASOPHIL(E) (SEE COLOR ATLAS)

d. Platelets (Thrombocytes)—irregularly shaped fragments of cytoplasm that break off from the megakaryocyte in the bone marrow.

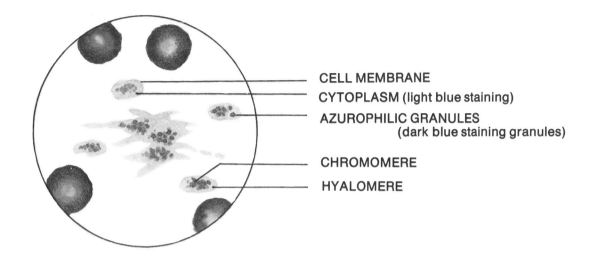

FIG. 3.12. PLATELETS (THROMBOCYTES) (SEE COLOR ATLAS)

The region of the platelet that contains the granules is known as the chromomere; the surrounding cytoplasm is the hyalomere.

2.   **Agranulocytes.—**

  a. **Lymphocyte.—**Small, medium and large size, the difference in size has to do with the amount of cytoplasm around the nucleus.

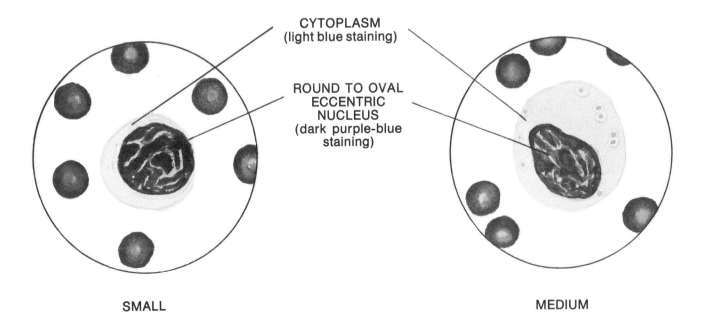

SMALL   MEDIUM

FIG. 3.13. LYMPHOCYTES—SMALL AND MEDIUM (SEE COLOR ATLAS)

The round to oval eccentric nucleus takes up most of the cell.

b. Monocyte.—Largest of the circulating blood cells. The monocyte is often irregularly shaped.

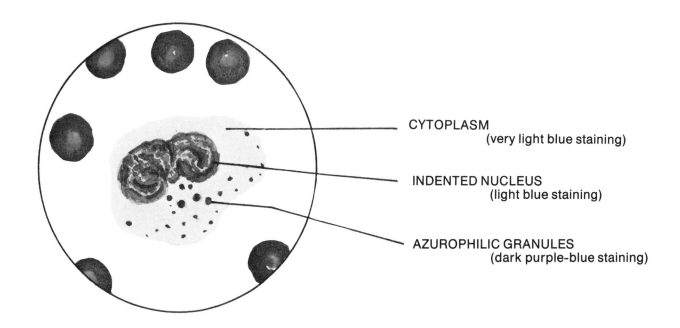

CYTOPLASM
(very light blue staining)

INDENTED NUCLEUS
(light blue staining)

AZUROPHILIC GRANULES
(dark purple-blue staining)

FIG. 3.14. MONOCYTE (SEE COLOR ATLAS)

The azurophilic granules found in the cytoplasm in the region of the indented nucleus is not a constant feature in all monocytes.

IV. COUNTING THE CELLS AND REPORTING THE COUNT

Once the white blood cells have been identified, the cells must be counted to obtain the differential white blood cell count.

A. Focusing Smear Under the Microscope

1. Use low power of the microscope to bring smear into focus; total magnification ca 100X. Focus with coarse adjustment.
2. The microscope's being parfocal, switch to the high power and focus sharply with <u>fine adjustment only</u>. Move smear to its thin end and locate one area where the red cells are evenly distributed, total magnification ca 400X.
3. Place a drop of immersion oil on the area of smear to be counted, switch to oil immersion lens, focus sharply with fine adjustment <u>only</u>, adjust light with iris diaphragm, total magnification ca 1000X.

B.   Movement of the Blood Smear

Begin at bottom of thin end of smear, scan the smears from lower edge to upper edge, then move slightly into thicker part of smear, scan from upper to lower edge, then move slightly into thicker part of smear and repeat. As you scan the smear in this pattern identify and count the white cells. This prescribed manner of counting allows you to count the cell only once.

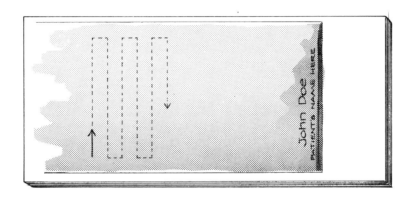

FIG. 3.15.   MOVEMENT OF SLIDE FOR DIFFERENTIAL

C.   Schilling Classification of White Cells

As you identify the white cells, count them on a differential laboratory counter or set up a sheet according to the Schilling classification (see Table 3.1). One hundred white cells are counted. After counting, record results accurately on the hemotology requisition slip. The normal percentages for the differential white cell count are given in Table 3.1. One should also examine red cells as differential proceeds.

TABLE 3.1

SCHILLING CLASSIFICATION (EXAMPLE)

Cells	Tally	No.	Normal %
Neutrophilic band cells	ЦНТ	5	2–6
Neutrophilic segmented cells		60	55–75
Lymphocytes	ЦНТ ЦНТ ЦНТ ЦНТ ЦНТ ЦНТ ЦНТ ЦНТ ЦНТ ЦНТ ЦНТ ЦНТ ЦНТ ЦНТ ЦНТ ЦНТ ЦНТ I	26	20–35
Monocytes	ЦНТ	5	2–6
Eosinophils	III	3	1–3
Basophils	I	1	0–1
Total		100	

If a Schilling count is not requested, the differential would not differentiate between "band cells" and "neutrophilic segmented cells."

D. Cells Reported as Part of the 100 Cell Count

Do not skip any cells; count all distorted cells which can be recognized, all overstained or understained cells which can be recognized.

E. Cells Reported But Not as Part of the 100 Cell Count

Report cells such as immature white cells, disintegrated cells, neutrophils with toxic granules, hypersegmented neutrophils, vacuolated cells and tissue cells.

F. Cells Not Reported as Part of 100 Cell Count

1. **Smudge Cells.**—Nucleus of ruptured white cell.

2. **Basket Cells.**—Net-like nucleus of a ruptured white cell. These last 2 types of cells should be reported if found in high numbers which indicate increased cellular fragility of these cells.

3. **Crescent Bodies.**—Remains of old red cells.

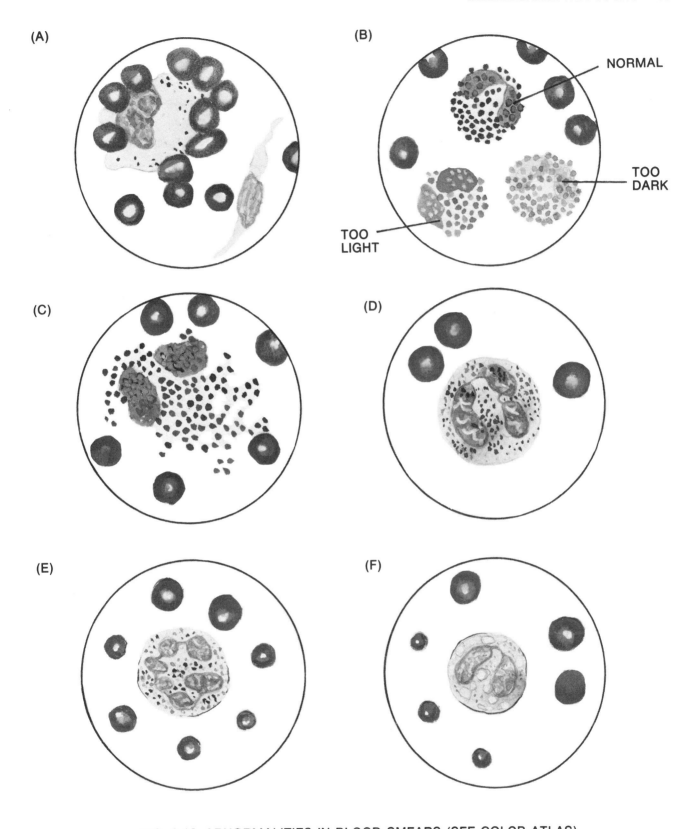

FIG. 3.16. ABNORMALITIES IN BLOOD SMEARS (SEE COLOR ATLAS)

(A) Lymphocytes showing distortion due to making smear.
(B) Poorly stained cells.
(C) Disintegrated cell.
(D) Neutrophil with toxic granulation.
(E) Hypersegmented neutrophil.
(F) Vacuolated neutrophil.

(A)

(B)

(C)

(D)

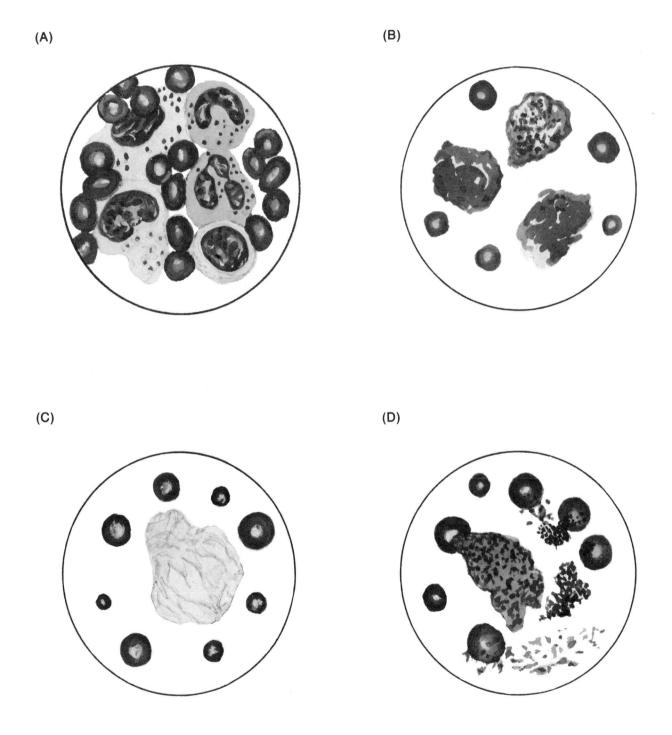

FIG. 3.17. ABNORMALITIES IN BLOOD SMEARS (SEE COLOR ATLAS)
(A) White cells at edge of smears.
(B) Smudge cells.
(C) Basket cell.
(D) Precipitated stain.

PROGRAMMED QUESTIONS

Cover answers with a piece of paper.   Answers appear at end of questions.

(1) What is one factor that determines thinness of the blood smear?
   (a) "Feathered" end extends to end of the slide
   (b) Time of application of stain
   (c) Angle of "spreader" slide
   (d) Using first drop of blood from the fingertip puncture

(2) What substance is used as a fixative in any staining procedures for the blood smear?
   (a) Methylene blue
   (b) Methyl alcohol
   (c) Phosphate buffer
   (d) Distilled water

(3) What should rise to the surface of staining solution if there is a proper mixing of stain and buffer in the Wright's staining procedure?
   (a) Metallic green sheen
   (b) Phosphate buffer
   (c) Eosin stain
   (d) None of the above

(4) How many lobes of the nucleus does the mature neutrophil usually exhibit?
   (a) 1–2
   (b) Band-shaped
   (c) 6–7
   (d) 3–5

(5) What is the prescribed manner of scanning the blood smear to count a differential WBC count?
   (a) Begin at thick end of smear and go to thin end
   (b) Begin at bottom margin of the smear, proceed to top margin and then go down, starting at thin end of smear
   (c) Move in any random manner
   (d) Begin at thin end of smear and proceed from center of smear toward the top and bottom margins

(6) In the Wright's staining procedure, if eosin dissociates too much and thus stains too brightly, the pH of the buffer is _____.
   (a) Too basic
   (b) Too acidic
   (c) Neutral
   (d) None of the above

(7) What is the normal lymphocyte percentage in a differential white cell count?
   (a) 1–3%
   (b) 60–75%
   (c) 20–35%
   (d) 2–10%

(8) What term describes a white cell in which the nucleus has ruptured?
   (a) Smudge cell
   (b) Crescent bodies
   (c) Band cell
   (d) Smear cell

(9) In what position is the "spreader" slide first placed before the smear is made?
   (a) On the drop of blood
   (b) Behind the drop of blood
   (c) Ahead of the drop(s) of blood
   (d) It makes no difference

(10) How is the "spreader" slide moved across the first slide in making a blood smear?
   (a) Pulling movement
   (b) Up and down movement
   (c) Swirling movement
   (d) Pushing movement

Answers

(1) c   (6) b
(2) b   (7) c
(3) a   (8) a
(4) d   (9) c
(5) b   (10) d

Hematocrit or
Packed Red Cell Volume

The hematocrit is estimated by centrifugation of anticoagulated whole blood to separate the cells from the plasma. The hematocrit is the volume of erythrocytes expressed as a percentage of the volume of whole blood. Hematocrit represents the concentration of the erythrocytes in the whole blood. In addition to volume of erythrocytes, one can obtain the height of "buffy" coat (white cells and platelets) and volume and appearance of the plasma. The hematocrit is the most reliable of all red cell measurements. The hematocrit, red cell count and hemoglobin estimation are directly related to each other. If one value is low, the other two values are usually low and vice versa.

I. NORMAL HEMATOCRIT VALUES

Men	47% ± 7%
Women	42% ± 5%
Average hematocrit for adults	42–45%
Children, 3 months–13 years	31–43%

II. CONDITIONS THAT CAUSE THE HEMATOCRIT TO VARY FROM NORMAL

A. High Hematocrits

1. **Polycythemia (Vera or Transitory).**—Hematocrit values are above normal when red cells are produced excessively.
2. **Dehydration**

B. Low Hematocrits

Hematocrit values below normal in:

1. **Anemia.**—Decreased red cell production.

2. **Leukemia.**—White cell production crowds out red cell production in the bone marrow.
3. **Excessive Fluid in the Blood (Hydremia).**—In this condition concentration of erythrocytes is low, but total mass of erythrocytes is not reduced.

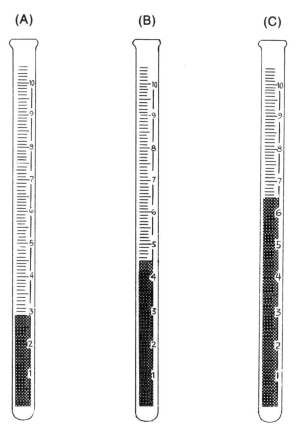

FIG. 4.1. VARIED HEMATOCRIT READINGS
(A) Low.
(B) Normal.
(C) High.

III. CALCULATING THE HEMATOCRIT

The hematocrit estimate is made by centrifuging a sample of anticoagulated blood and calculating the percent volume occupied by the packed red cells.

$$\text{Hematocrit (\%)} = \frac{\text{(height of red cell column in cm)}}{\text{(height of whole blood in cm)}} \times 100$$

Example: Height of red cell column   4.5 cm
             Height of whole blood   10.0 cm

$$\text{Hematocrit (\%)} = \frac{4.5\ \text{cm}}{10\ \text{cm}} \times 100$$
$$0.45 \times 100 = 45\%$$

IV.MACRO-HEMATOCRIT ESTIMATION— WINTROBE METHOD ON VENOUS BLOOD

A. Materials

1. Anticoagulated tube blood taken from venipuncture. The anticoagulant could be either heparin, oxalate or EDTA.
2. Disposable Wintrobe tubes—narrow, thick-walled, uniform bore tubes, with flattened bottom. The right side of the tube is graduated for hematocrit from 0–10 cm from bottom to top.
3. Disposable "Wintrobe" pipette with attached rubber bulb. Pipette must reach bottom of the Wintrobe tube.
4. Bench model centrifuge with bucket head.

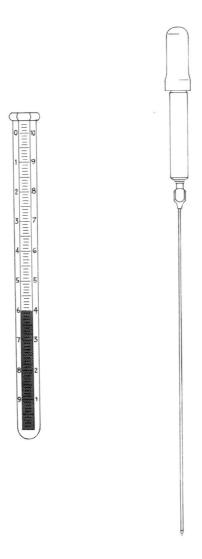

FIG. 4.2. WINTROBE TUBE AND PIPETTE

B. Method

1. **Suspend Blood Cells.—**Mix tube of blood thoroughly by slowly inverting tube. If blood is at room temperature invert 10–12 times; if blood is cold allow blood to return to room temperature, invert 10–20 times slowly.

2. **Filling "Wintrobe" Pipette with Blood.—**

   a. Attach rubber bulb to end of "Wintrobe" pipette. Place bulb halfway on end of pipette.
   b. Exclude air from pipette by pressing on rubber bulb.
   c. Gradually release pressure on the bulb and allow blood to be drawn into the pipette about halfway.

3. **Filling Wintrobe Tube with Blood.—**

   a. Place "Wintrobe" pipette filled with blood into bottom of Wintrobe tube.
   b. Keep Wintrobe tube on a slant, press rubber bulb of the pipette continuously so the blood flows out of the pipette.

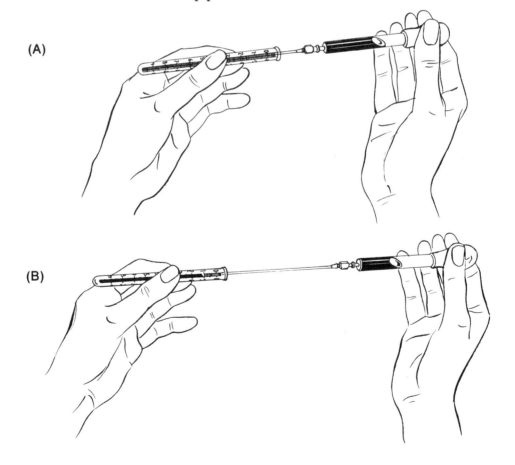

FIG. 4.3. FILLING WINTROBE TUBE
(A) Needle at bottom of tube.
(B) Expelling blood while withdrawing needle.

    c. Fill Wintrobe tube from the bottom. As blood comes out, slowly withdraw the pipette, but continue pressure on the rubber bulb of the pipette so as to exclude air bubbles. Try to keep the tip of the pipette under the rising column of blood to avoid foaming.

    d. Fill Wintrobe tube to the 10 cm mark exactly. Fill a second tube to balance the centrifuge. Label tubes with patient's number or initials.

4. Centrifugation.—

    a. Place Wintrobe tubes in opposite cups of the centrifuge for balance. Check to see if cups have rubber bumpers on the bottom.

    b. Turn centrifuge on and slowly bring up to full speed. Operate at full speed (about 3000 rpm) for 30 min.

5. Reading the Hematocrit and Reporting the Results.—

    a. Read hematocrit or packed red cell volume directly off the calibration on the right side of the Wintrobe tube. Do not include the "buffy" coat in your reading.

    b. Report results on the hematology requisition slip to include name of method and percentage volume of packed red cells of the whole blood.

V. MICRO-CAPILLARY HEMATOCRIT ESTIMATION

A. Materials

    1.   Capillary blood or venipuncture blood
    2.   Capillary tubes (75 mm long × 1.1–1.2 mm in diameter)—heparinized for capillary blood or plain for venipuncture blood
    3.   Sealing clay for capillary tubes
    4.   Micro-hematocrit centrifuge
    5.   Micro-hematocrit tube reader and card reader

B. Method

1. Fingertip Puncture.—If using fingertip capillary blood, make a finger puncture and wipe away the first two drops of blood. This is necessary to ensure free-flowing blood.

2. Filling Capillary Tubes and Sealing Off the Tubes.—

    a. Put one end of a heparinized capillary tube into the drop of blood. Tilt other end downward so blood flows into the tube. Fill two capillary tubes 3/4 full of blood. If you get air in the column of blood it is not significant, since air gap will disappear on centrifugation. Mix by tilting left and right and by rolling capillary tube between hands (see Fig. 4.5).

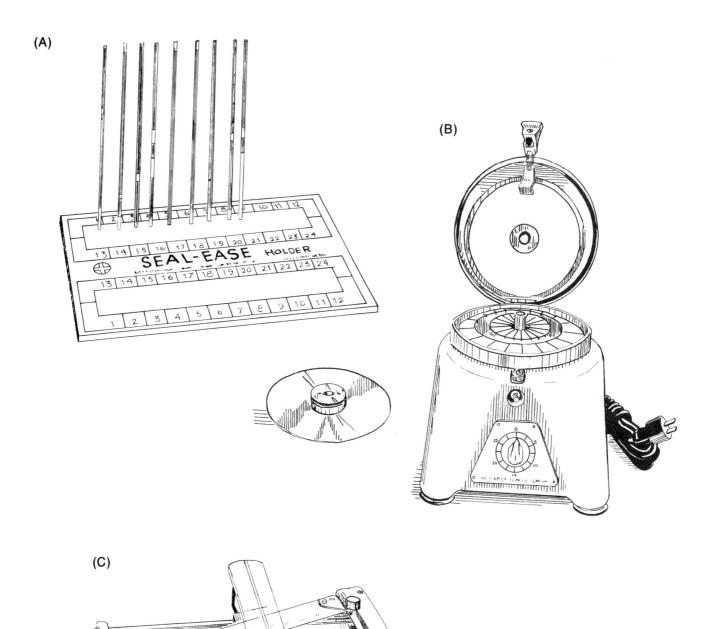

FIG. 4.4.   MICRO-HEMATOCRIT APPARATUS
(A) Capillary tubes and sealing clay.
(B) Centrifuge.
(C) Micro-hematocrit tube reader.

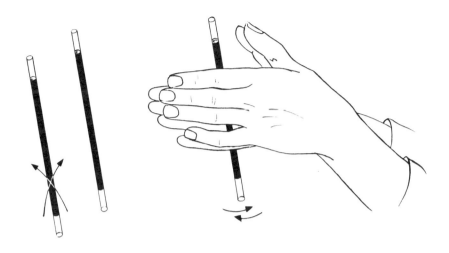

FIG. 4.5. MIXING OF BLOOD IN CAPILLARY TUBE

b. Seal off one end of capillary tube by sticking the end into sealing clay. Twist tube and remove a plug of clay. The clay plug should form a straight edge across bottom of column of blood.

3. Centrifugation.—

a. Place capillary tubes into opposite radial grooves of the micro-hematocrit centrifuge head with sealed ends contacting the rubber gasket. Remember number of grooves in which you placed the capillary tubes. Put cover on head and tighten. Spin centrifuge head by hand to make certain capillary tubes contact rubber gasket.

b. Close lid of centrifuge, turn centrifuge on, spin for 10 min. The micro-hematocrit centrifuge has no speed control. When turned on it operates at full speed (10,000–12,000 rpm). In some laboratories time of centrifugation is between 3–5 min.

4. Reading the Hematocrit on the Micro-hematocrit "Readers" and Reporting the Results.—Since the capillary tubes are not graduated, the packed red cell volume in the capillary tube is read by either the micro-hematocrit tube reader or card reader. (Actually a ruler can also be used.)

a. Micro-hematocrit Tube Reader.—

(1) Place capillary tube in groove in plastic holder, slide capillary tube to bottom of holder and line up the bottom of the packed red cells with the bottom edge of the tube reader bar or ruler.

(2) Move plastic holder until the meniscus of plasma in the capillary tube coincides with 100 mm mark on the reader bar.

(3) Tighten the knob at the end of the reader bar.

(4) Slide plastic holder until reader bar coincides with line separating packed red cells from the plasma.

(5) Read percentage of packed red cells or hematocrit directly off the reader bar.

(6) Report the method, i.e., micro-capillary hematocrit, and percentage volume of packed red cells of whole blood.

b. Micro-hematocrit Card Reader.—See directions on the card.

VI. SOURCES OF ERROR IN HEMATOCRIT

A. Centrifugation—Inadequate centrifugation: centrifugation must be of adequate speed and duration of time. The red cells must be packed so that additional centrifugation will not reduce the packed red cell volume any further. High hematocrits need higher centrifugal force to spin cells down than do low hematocrits.

B. Trapping of leukocytes, platelets and plasma in between the red cells is normally insignificant if centrifugation is of adequate speed and duration, but if there is low centrifugal force larger amounts are trapped. Amounts of these components trapped is larger in high hematocrits compared to low hematocrits and larger in the macro method than in the micro method.

C. Failure to mix tube blood adequately before using with the result that the cells are not fully suspended is a major source of error in the macro method.

D. Leaking of blood from sealed end of capillary tube due to improper sealing of the sealing clay.

E. Improper reading of the level of the red cells, i.e., reading of the "buffy" coat as part of the red cell volume.

F. Excessive anticoagulant causes red cells to shrink and lowers hematocrit reading.

G. Interior diameter of capillary tubes not constant; leads to inaccurate hematocrits.

VII. ADVANTAGES OF MICRO-CAPILLARY METHOD

A. Time of centrifugation. Micro—10 min or less versus macro—30 min

B. Less error due to trapping of leukocytes, platelets and plasma due to smaller volume used

C. Ease of filling capillary tubes

D. Need for a small volume of blood

E. Duplicate determinations easy to obtain—only major precaution is to use free-flowing blood.

PROGRAMMED QUESTIONS

Cover answers with a piece of paper.   Answers appear at end of questions.

(1) The percent concentration of erythrocytes in the whole blood expresses _____.
   (a) Hemoglobin value
   (b) Hematocrit
   (c) RBC count
   (d) Sedimentation rate

(2) Choose from the following a condition causing a high hematocrit.
   (a) Hydremia
   (b) Leukemia
   (c) Leakage of blood from capillary tube
   (d) Low centrifugal force

(3) What must you do to prevent air bubbles from entering the column of blood when filling the Wintrobe tube for a macro-hematocrit?
   (a) Keep continual pressure on rubber bulb of Wintrobe pipette
   (b) Gradually release pressure on rubber bulb on Wintrobe pipette
   (c) Operate centrifuge at adequate speed on duration
   (d) None of the above

(4) To read the height of the erythrocyte column in the micro-hematocrit method, _____.
   (a) Line up the top of the erythrocyte column to the 100 mm mark on the tube reader bar or ruler
   (b) Line up the bottom of the erythrocyte column to the bottom edge of the tube reader bar or ruler
   (c) Line up the "buffy" coat with the bottom edge of the tube reader bar or ruler
   (d) Read the marking on the right side of the capillary tube

(5) What are two advantages of the micro-capillary hematocrit method?
   (a) Need small volume; time of centrifugation 30 min
   (b) Duplicate determinations easy to obtain; excessive anticoagulant does not affect hematocrit reading
   (c) Time of centrifugation short; need only a small volume of blood
   (d) Interior diameter of capillary tube does not have to be constant; ease in filling capillary tube

(6) What is the normal hematocrit reading for women?
   (a) 37–47%
   (b) 31–35%
   (c) 40–54%
   (d) 60–75%

(7) Which hematological procedure uses heparinized capillary tubes?
   (a) Macro-hematocrit
   (b) Capillary coagulation tube
   (c) Cyanmethemoglobin
   (d) Micro-hematocrit

(8) In the micro-hematocrit method, where is the 100 mm mark of the reader bar set in the micro-hematocrit tube reader?
   (a) At the "buffy" coat
   (b) At meniscus of the plasma
   (c) At the height of the red cell column
   (d) At the junction of the red cell column and the clay plug

(9) Approximately how many times should tube blood be inverted before use after blood has been removed from the refrigerator and returned to room temperature?
(a) 10–20 times
(b) 75–100 times
(c) 10–50 times
(d) It does not matter

(10) Which is <u>not</u> a source of error in the micro-capillary hematocrit procedure?
(a) Use of freshly drawn blood
(b) Air bubbles in column of blood
(c) Excessive anticoagulant
(d) Partially clotted blood

Answers

(1) b
(2) d
(3) a
(4) b
(5) c

(6) a
(7) d
(8) b
(9) a
(10) a or b

Hemocytometry—The White and Red Blood Cell Count

I. PRINCIPLES OF HEMOCYTOMETRY

Hematological diagnostic tests are divided into two groups:

A. Chemical Tests

Chemical tests are concerned with hemoglobin and biochemical measurements on the blood cells.

B. Morphological Tests

1. **Qualitative Tests.**—Qualitative tests are concerned with the appearance of red and white cells in a stained blood smear.

2. **Quantitative Tests.**—Quantitative tests are concerned with counting and calculating the total number of red cells, white cells and platelets in a specific volume of blood. Hemocytometry deals with the quantitative tests.

   The principle of hemocytometry consists of making an accurate dilution of a measured quantity of blood with diluting fluid. A specific volume of the diluted blood is placed in a counting chamber and a number of cells in this volume is counted. From this count, the number of cells/mm^3 of blood is calculated and reported.

II. HEMOCYTOMETRY APPARATUS FOR MANUAL COUNTING

The basic apparatus used in manual quantitative studies of the blood cells is the hemocytometer kit. It consists of the white and red cell diluting pipettes and the counting chamber or hemocytometer slide.

A. Diluting Pipettes

The diluting pipettes consist of a relatively long capillary tube containing equal divisions marked prominently at the 0.5 and 1 mark. Above the mixing bulb is a short capillary tube marked 11 on the white cell pipette and 101 on the red cell pipette. All graduation markings are arbitrary as they give the ratio of the resultant dilution. They do not indicate the actual cubic millimeters of blood and diluting fluid taken up.

1. **Routine White Cell Dilution.**—The white cell pipette has a small mixing bulb with a white bead. When blood is drawn to the 0.5 mark <u>exactly</u> and diluted with white cell diluting fluid to the 11 mark, the dilution is 1 to 20 <u>and the</u> dilution factor is 20.

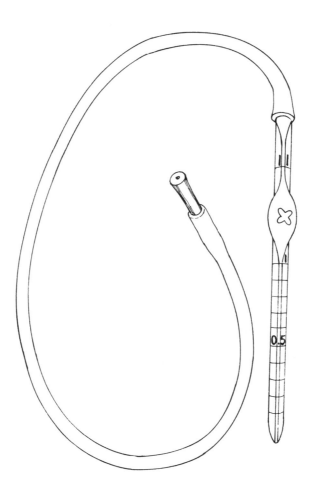

FIG. 5.1.   WHITE CELL PIPETTE AND ASPIRATOR

2. **Routine Red Cell Dilution.**—The red cell pipette has a large mixing bulb with a red bead. When blood is drawn to the 0.5 mark <u>exactly</u> and diluted with red cell diluting fluid to the 101 mark, the dilution is 1 to 200 <u>and the</u> dilution factor is 200.

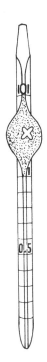

FIG. 5.2. RED CELL PIPETTE (FILLED)

No air bubbles should be present in the column of blood or after the dilution fluid is added.

If the dilutions are properly made, all blood cells in the capillary of the pipette are washed into the mixing bulb and the capillary of the pipette should contain only diluting fluid. The cell-free fluid is not included in the dilution of the cells, since it is expelled before the blood cells charge the counting chamber.

B. Neubauer Counting Chamber

The Neubauer counting chamber is a bright line hemocytometer. The rulings on the chamber are distinct, since they are metallically coated. The hemocytometer slide consists of a central platform containing 2 counting chambers separated by a groove. The depth of the counting chamber is 0.1 mm, as the central platform is 0.1 mm lower than the lateral platforms on which the cover glass rests.

1. **White Cell Sections.**—Each counting chamber consists of a ruled square containing nine 1 mm^2 sections. The 4 corner squares are used for the white cell count (marked W in Fig. 5.4). The total volume held in the 4 white cell corner sections is 0.4 mm^3.

depth of counting chamber		area of each white cell square		number of squares counted		total volume
0.1 mm	$\times$	1 mm^2	$\times$	4	$=$	0.4 mm^3

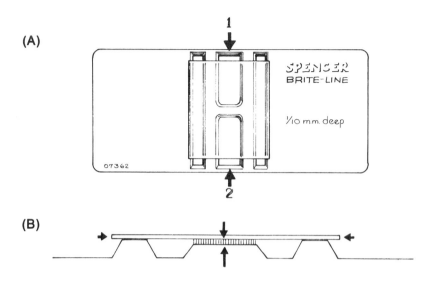

FIG. 5.3. HEMOCYTOMETER SLIDE WITH COVER GLASS
(A) Surface view.
(B) Side view (greatly enlarged).

2. **Red Cell Sections.**—The central square of the counting chamber is used for the red cell count. This square is divided into 25 smaller squares. As a rule 5 of these smaller squares are used for the red cell count, the 4 corner squares and the central square. The area of each of these squares is 0.04 mm². The total volume held in the 5 red cell sections is 0.02 mm³.

depth of   area of each   number of
counting chamber × red cell square × squares counted = total volume

0.1 mm   ×   0.04 mm²   ×   5   =   0.02 mm³

C. Diluting Fluids

1. **Red Cell Diluting Fluids.**—The red cell diluting fluids are isotonic to that of the red cells to prevent hemolysis (swelling and bursting) or crenation (shrinkage). The diluting fluids also "fix" the cells to preserve them and prevent agglutination of the red cells. Two commonly used red cell diluting fluids are:

a. Hayem's solution which consists of mercuric chloride ($HgCl_2$), NaCl, Na_2SO_4 and H_2O

b. Gower's solution which consists of Na_2SO_4, acetic acid (HAc) and H_2O.

Gower's solution is superior to Hayem's solution, since it prevents rouleaux formation.

2. **White Cell Diluting Fluids.**—The purpose of the white cell diluting fluid is to hemolyze the red cells so they will not obscure the white cells. Two commonly used white cell diluting fluids are:

a. 2% Acetic acid (most popular)

b. 1% (0.1N) HCl

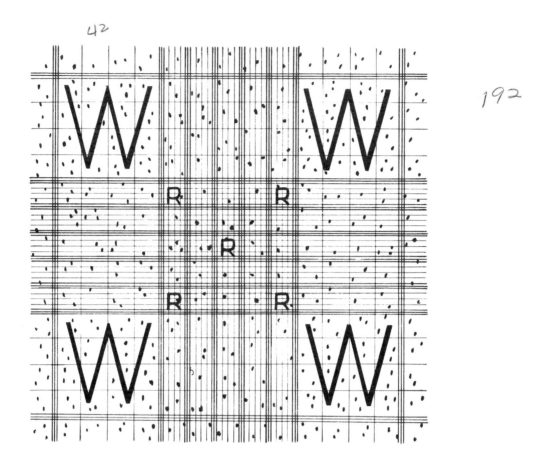

FIG. 5.4. COUNTING CHAMBER SHOWING POSITION OF THE WHITE AND RED CELL SECTIONS FOR COUNTING OF WHITE AND RED CELLS

III. WITHDRAWAL OF THE BLOOD SAMPLE

Blood from a fingertip puncture or anticoagulated venipuncture blood can be used. If blood is not anticoagulated, all steps must be rapidly performed in withdrawal of the blood sample in order to prevent coagulation.

A. Assemble all equipment needed for fingertip puncture. Loosen or remove caps on diluting fluid bottles before starting the withdrawal of the blood sample. Make sure all fluids are clean and fresh.

B. Fingertip puncture is made in the usual manner. The first drop of blood is wiped off.

C. The pipette tip is loosely immersed in the drop of blood, with pipette held on a slant and with graduation marks visible. The blood is drawn up exactly, if possible, to the 0.5 mark in both red and white cell pipettes. The drop of blood must be large enough; otherwise air bubbles will be drawn into the pipette. Beginning students may have difficulty in reaching the line exactly! If this occurs, draw blood above the 0.5 mark (see Section E).

D. Air bubbles in the pipette can be due to:
    1. Drop of blood too small
    2. Tip of pipette not fully immersed in drop of blood

3. Tip of pipette broken
4. Pipette not dry and clean

E. Pipetting greatly beyond the 0.5 mark: Another problem to consider is not to have the column of blood rise too greatly beyond the 0.5 mark. If blood is only slightly above the mark, tease blood out to the mark by touching tip of pipette to gauze pad. If there is a large excess of blood above the mark, repeat procedure with a dry, clean pipette, since enough blood will remain adhering to the inside of the pipette to introduce a significant error. Accuracy and precision are important in this part of the procedure since any error is magnified 200 times for red cell count and 20 times for white cell count on dilution with the diluting fluids.

IV. DILUTION OF THE BLOOD SAMPLE AND MIXING OF BLOOD WITH DILUTING FLUIDS

A. Filling Pipette with Diluting Fluids

Make sure caps on diluting fluid bottles are loosened or removed. With tongue over hole in the mouthpiece, place tip of pipette into the diluting fluid. Then quickly draw up the diluting fluid to the 11 mark for the white cell dilution and 101 mark for red cell dilution. Hold pipette in diluting fluid on a slant to avoid getting air bubbles in the bulb of the pipette. Rotate pipette as diluting fluid is being drawn up to ensure mixing and to prevent coagulation. When bulb of pipette is almost full, raise pipette to vertical position. As the top mark of the pipette is approached, either place tongue over hole in the mouthpiece or pinch the aspirator tubing over the top of the pipette to stop at the proper diluting line. Then withdraw pipette from diluting fluid; place pipette in horizontal position.

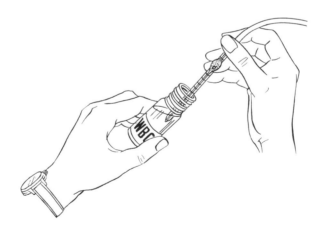

FIG. 5.5.   POSITION FOR HOLDING DILUTING FLUID BOTTLE AND PIPETTE

B. Removal of Aspirator Tubing

With the pipette horizontal, place one finger over tip of pipette and with other hand disconnect tubing. If finger is not over tip of pipette, fluid will squirt out as you disconnect aspirator.

C. Mixing Blood with Diluting Fluid in the Pipette

Place thumb and forefinger over ends of pipette. Hand-shake pipette end to end and rotate between hands for 10 sec to prevent blood coagulation. A commercial pipette closure may be applied if so desired.

1. **Hand-shaking.**—Move pipette back and forth by flicking wrist up and down while arm does not move and by keeping pipette parallel to the floor. Shake pipettes vigorously for 3–5 min.

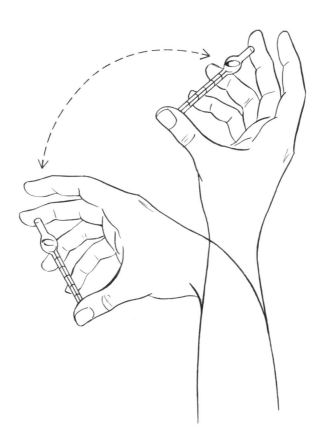

FIG. 5.6.   METHOD FOR HAND-SHAKING PIPETTE

2. **Automatic Shaking.**—After hand-shaking for 10 sec, place pipettes into a mechanical shaker for 45 sec. Pipette closures may be placed over ends of the pipettes.

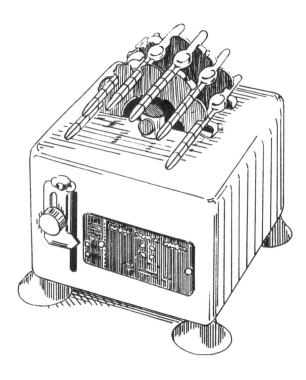

FIG. 5.7.   AUTOMATIC YANKEE SHAKER

V. CHARGING THE COUNTING CHAMBERS

A. Cleaning Chamber and Cover Glass, and Cover Glass Placement

Clean counting chamber and ground glass cover slip with lens paper or gauze. Place cover glass on top of counting chamber as illustrated in Fig. 5.3.

B. Discarding the First Drops of Diluting Fluid

After shaking the pipettes, discard the first 3 to 4 drops of diluting fluid in the capillary portion of the pipette into a tissue or gauze pad. Theoretically, this should be cell-free fluid.

C. Charging the Chambers

With the name of the manufacturer of the counting chamber to your right, charge the upper chamber with white cells and the lower chamber with red cells.

The chambers are charged in the following manner. The pipette is held on a slant with the tip of the pipette placed against the edge of the cover glass. The fluid enters the chamber in a controlled manner by capillary attraction and pressure from the index finger on the top of the pipette. The cover glass should not be moved during filling. If it has that tendency, gently hold it in place as indicated in Fig. 5.8. Permit just enough fluid to entirely fill the space beneath the cover glass of one chamber. Excess fluid raises the cover glass, changes the volume and increases the cell count. If the chamber has been overcharged, or excess fluid is in the well, the chamber may be recharged or excess can be removed by briefly touching tip of gauze pad to excess. Your instructor may suggest other techniques.

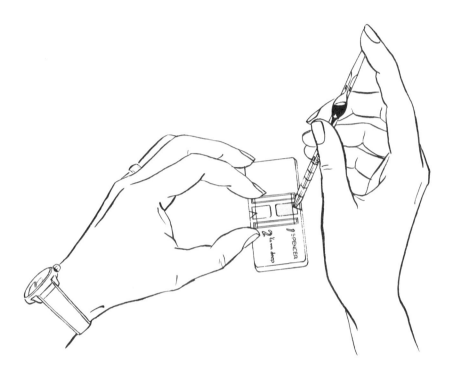

FIG. 5.8. CHARGING THE COUNTING CHAMBER

The same procedure is used to charge the WBC chamber and the RBC chamber. Traditionally the upper chamber is charged with WBC; the lower with RBC. This is not of great importance since both chambers have the same rulings.

D. Criteria of Properly Charged Chambers

A properly filled chamber has the fluid entirely filling the space beneath the cover glass. None of the fluid is running over into the groove and there are no air bubbles. If these conditions are not met, clean and recharge the counting chambers. If the time lapse between filling and charging the chambers is over 2 min, reshake pipettes by hand or on the mechanical shaker as described previously, discard the first 3 to 4 drops, then recharge chambers. The reshaking assures that the cells are well suspended before recharging the chambers.

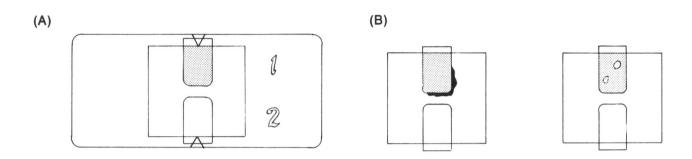

FIG. 5.9.   (A) PROPERLY CHARGED COUNTING CHAMBER
(B) IMPROPERLY CHARGED COUNTING CHAMBER

VI. COUNTING THE CELLS AND MAKING THE CALCULATIONS

Before counting the cells, allow cells about 1 to 3 min to settle on the counting chamber. Count the white cells first, since they (being larger) will settle more rapidly than red cells.

A. White Cells

1.   **Counting the Cells.—**

a. **Normal Values for the White Cell Count.—**

Adult (no sex difference)	5000–10,000/mm^3 of blood
Children about 1 year	8000–15,000/mm^3 of blood
Infants at birth	10,000–25,000/mm^3 of blood

b. **Locating the Rulings of the White Cell Counting Chamber.—**Under the scanning objective of the microscope, focus sharply on the well of the counting chamber, then move the stage of the microscope until the rulings of the counting chamber are seen; sharpen the focus. Under this magnification, the entire ruled area can be observed, with the white cells' appearing as black, glistening, refractile dots when the iris diaphragm is used to cut down the light.

c. **Check for a Good Distribution of White Cells.—**Before beginning the count, check for a good distribution of cells. The white cells should be almost evenly distributed throughout the counting chamber. If distribution is poor, clean chamber, reshake white cell pipette, discard first 3 to 4 drops, and recharge the chamber.

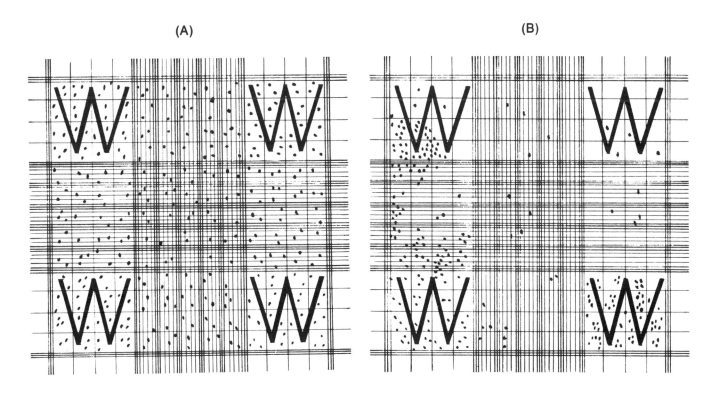

(A)   (B)

FIG. 5.10.   (A) GOOD VERSUS (B) BAD DISTRIBUTION OF WHITE CELLS

d. Lens Under Which Cells Are Counted, and Making the Count.—If distribution of cells is good, switch to the low power lens. The white cells are counted in the 4 corner squares, called the "W" sections. Only one entire W section can be observed through the low power objective of the microscope. The first W section is in the upper left corner. There should be no squares directly above it and directly to the left of it. The second W section is in the upper right corner. The third and fourth W sections are in the lower right and left corners respectively.

Start the count in the upper left small square of each W section and count the cells in the 16 small squares of each W section. In the first or top row, proceed from left to right; second row to the left; third row to the right; fourth row to the left. If a cell lies on a boundary line of a square, in order to count the cell once, the rules are:

(1)   Count those cells on the upper and left boundary lines.
(2)   Do not count those cells lying on the right and lower boundary lines.

If the white cell distribution is good, the count for any W section should not vary by more than 10 cells/W section. If variation is greater than that, an erroneous white cell count could be expected. Clean and recharge the chamber, and repeat the count.

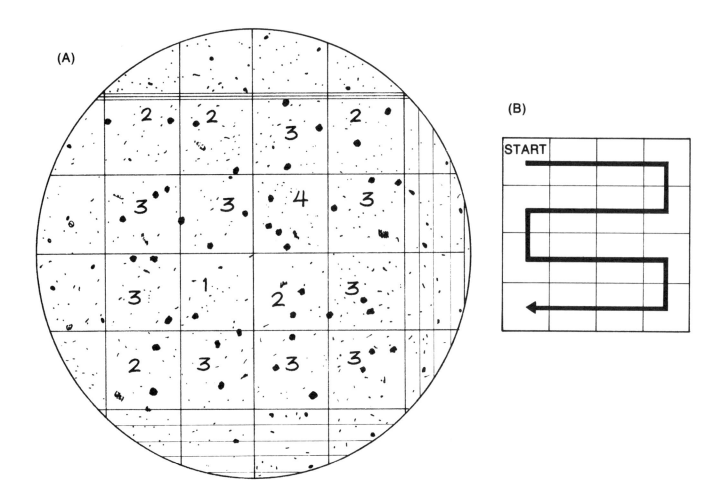

FIG. 5.11.   COUNTING THE CELLS IN THE "W" SECTION
(A) Microscopic view of white cells in the W section.
(B) Procedure for counting white cells.

2.   **Making the Calculations.**—The white cell count is reported as the number of white cells/mm^3 of <u>undiluted</u> blood. Since the blood was diluted and the cells were counted in a volume less than 1.0 mm^3, the number of cells counted must be multiplied by 2 correction factors.

a.   **Dilution Correction Factor.**—To compensate for dilution of the blood, the white cell dilution correction factor is 20, as the blood was diluted 20 times in the pipette.

b.   **Volume Correction Factor.**—To compensate for volume in which the white cells were counted, the volume correction factor is 2.5.

$$\text{volume correction factor} = \frac{\text{volume in which white cells are reported}}{\text{volume in which white cells are counted}} = \frac{1.0 \text{ mm}^3}{0.4 \text{ mm}^3} = 2.5$$

c. **Calculation of Number of WBC/mm³ of Blood.**—When total number of cells in the 4 W sections are multiplied by the two correction factors, the WBC/mm³ of blood is obtained.

$$\begin{array}{c}\text{number of white} \\ \text{cells counted} \\ \text{in 4 W sections}\end{array} \times \begin{array}{c}\text{dilution} \\ \text{correction} \\ \text{factor}\end{array} \times \begin{array}{c}\text{volume} \\ \text{correction} \\ \text{factor}\end{array} = \frac{\text{number of WBC}}{\text{mm}^3 \text{ of blood}}$$

Example: 100 $\times$ 20 $\times$ 2.5 $=$ 5000

The combined <u>normal</u> white cell correction factor (20 × 2.5) is 50, since dilution and volume correction factors are usually constant. The combined correction factor multiplied by the number of white cells counted in the 4 W sections gives the WBC/mm³ of blood, i.e., WBC counted in 4 sections times 50 equals WBC/mm³.

B. Red Cells

1. **Counting the Cells.—**

   a. **Normal Values for the Red Cell Count.—**

   Adult (sex difference)
Males	4.5–6.0 million/mm³ of blood
Females	4.0–5.5 million/mm³ of blood
Average adult values	4.0–6.0 million/mm³ of blood
Children	3.5–4.3 million/mm³ of blood
Infants	5.0–6.5 million/mm³ of blood

   b. **Locating the Rulings of the Red Cell Counting Chamber.**—Once count of WBC has been done under low power, move stage to other chamber. RBC square should be in focus under low power. The entire central square can be observed under low power of the microscope; sharpen the focus. The red cells appear as biconcave disks and are counted in the central square. You might also notice debris in the diluting fluid.

   c. **Check for a Good Distribution of Red Cells.**—Before beginning the count, check for a good distribution of cells. The red cells should be practically evenly distributed throughout the counting chamber. If the distribution is poor, clean chamber, reshake red cell pipette, discard first 3 to 4 drops, and recharge the chamber.

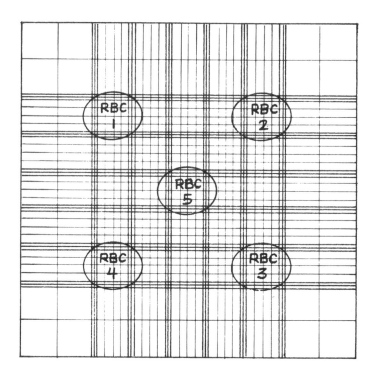

FIG. 5.12.   CENTRAL SQUARE OF COUNTING CHAMBER SHOWING WHERE
RED CELLS ARE TO BE COUNTED

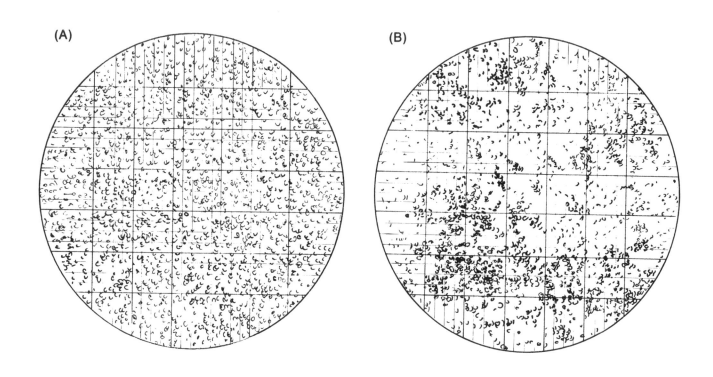

FIG. 5.13.   (A) GOOD VERSUS (B) BAD DISTRIBUTION OF RED CELLS

d. Lens Under Which Cells Are Counted, and Making the Count.—If distribution of cells is good, switch to high dry objective. Under this magnification, only one red (R) section can be seen. Each R section is bounded on all sides by double or triple lines and is composed of 16 smaller squares.

In making a normal red cell count, the cells in the four corner R sections and middle R section are counted (see Fig. 5.12). Begin the count in the first R section which is the upper left square. This section can be identified, as there is an absence of cross lines above and to the left of the section. Within the first R section, start in the upper left small square and count all the red cells in the 16 smaller squares of this R section. Proceed in the first or top row from left to right; second row to the left; third row to the right; fourth row to the left. In order to count the cell only once, in each square count cells which touch any upper and left boundary lines and do not count cells touching any lower and right boundary lines. Proceed to count the cells in the second, third, fourth and fifth R sections as described for the first. To find the fifth R section, after the cells of the fourth R section are counted, move the chamber 2 sections up and 2 sections to the right. The fifth R section is bounded on all sides by double or triple crossed lines. The total number of red cells normally counted in the 5 R sections is about 500. If distribution of red cells is good, the red cell count for each R section should not vary by more than 10.

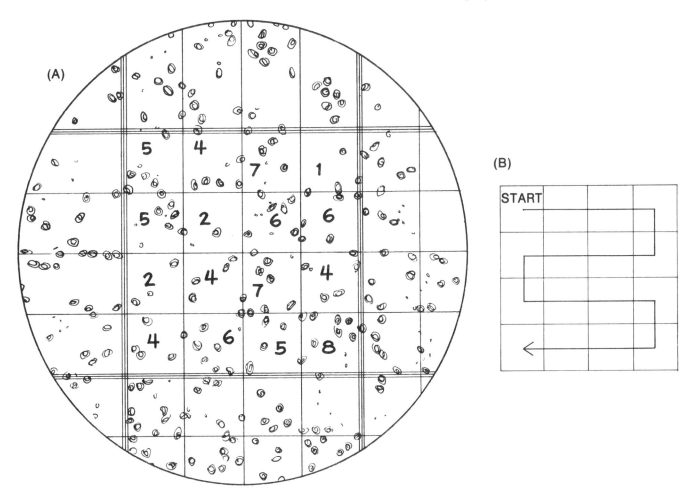

FIG. 5.14.   COUNTING THE CELLS IN THE "R" SECTION
(A) Microscopic view of red cells in the R section.
(B) Procedure for counting red cells.

2. **Making the Calculations.**—The red cell count is reported as the number of red cells/mm^3 of <u>undiluted</u> blood. Since the blood was diluted and cells were counted in a volume less than 1.0 mm^3, the number of cells counted must be multiplied by two correction factors.

a. **Dilution Correction Factor.**—To compensate for the dilution of the blood, the red cell dilution correction factor is 200, as the blood was diluted 200 times in the pipette.

b. **Volume Correction Factor.**—To compensate for the volume in which the red cells were counted, the volume correction factor is 50.

$$\text{volume correction factor} \ = \ \frac{\begin{array}{c}\text{volume in which red}\\ \text{cells are reported}\end{array}}{\begin{array}{c}\text{volume in which red}\\ \text{cells are counted}\end{array}} \ = \ \frac{1.0 \text{ mm}^3}{0.02 \text{ mm}^3} \ = \ 50$$

c. **Calculation of Number of RBC/mm³ of Blood.**—When total number of cells in the 5 R sections are multiplied by the two correction factors, the RBC/mm^3 of blood is obtained.

$$\begin{array}{c}\text{number of red}\\ \text{cells counted in}\\ \text{5 R sections}\end{array} \times \begin{array}{c}\text{dilution}\\ \text{correction}\\ \text{factor}\end{array} \times \begin{array}{c}\text{volume}\\ \text{correction}\\ \text{factor}\end{array} = \frac{\text{number of RBC}}{\text{mm}^3 \text{ of blood}}$$

$$500 \quad \times \quad 200 \quad \times \quad 50 \quad = \quad 5{,}000{,}000$$

The combined normal red cell correction factor (200 × 50) is 10,000 since dilution and volume correction factors are usually constant. The combined correction factor, multiplied by the number of cells counted in the 5 R sections gives the RBC/mm^3 of blood.

Another way of calculating red cells in 1.0 mm^3 of blood is to add 4 zeros to the total number of cells counted in the 5 R sections.

$$500 + 0000 = 5{,}000{,}000 \text{ RBC/mm}^3 \text{ of blood}$$

The 4 zeros are from the 10,000 (or 10^4) which is the combined normal dilution and correction factors for red cells.

VII. CORRECTION OF TOTAL WHITE CELL COUNT FOR NUCLEATED RED CELLS

If there are nucleated red cells (metarubricytes) in the blood, they are not hemolyzed by the white cell diluting fluids. If these cells were in high number, they would be counted as white cells and would contribute to an erroneous high white cell count, which would have to be corrected. If one finds a large number of nucleated red cells on examination of the blood smear during a white cell differential count, a correction in the total white cell count has to be made by use of the following formula.

$$\text{corrected white cell count} = \text{uncorrected white cell count} \times \frac{100}{(100 + x)}$$

100 = white cells counted in the differential white cell count

x = number of nucleated red cells counted while performing the 100 white cell differential count

Example:

white cell count = 15,000/mm³ of blood

x = 50 nucleated red cells seen on a white cell differential count

$$\text{correct white cell count} = 15,000 \times \frac{100}{(100 + 50)}$$

$$= 15,000 \times \frac{100}{150}$$

$$= 15,000 \times \frac{2}{3}$$

corrected white cell count = 10,000/mm³ of blood

VIII. CORRELATION OF THE DIFFERENTIAL COUNT WITH TOTAL WHITE CELL COUNT

After you have performed many total white cell counts and differential counts on adults, you will come to expect a certain type of differential count relative to the total white cell count. A high total white cell count should be accompanied by a differential count demonstrating a high neutrophil count and a low lymphocyte count. A low total white cell count should be accompanied by a relatively high lymphocyte count and low neutrophil count on the differential. In infants and preschool children there is always a high lymphocyte count compared to neutrophil count on the differential, no matter what the total white cell count may be.

IX.   MAJOR SOURCES OF ERROR IN WHITE AND RED CELL COUNTS

A. Failure to have blood exactly on the 0.5 mark of the pipette.

B. Failure to dilute the cells accurately to the 11 and 101 marks of the pipettes.

C. Failure to shake the pipette thoroughly—inadequate and improper shaking.

D. Failure to discard the first 3 to 4 drops from the pipette before filling the chamber.

E. Failure to properly charge the counting chamber—overflowing or air bubbles in counting chamber.

F. Slowness in manipulation; allowing blood to clot.

G. Touching cover glass with microscope objective, causing pressure and reducing depth of counting chamber.

H. Presence of yeast or dirt in diluting fluid, thus mistaking specks for cells.

I. Dirty or greasy apparatus.

J. Failure to wipe excess blood from sides and tip of pipette—air bubbles in column of blood.

K. Using wet, unclean or broken pipettes; tip of pipette must not be chipped.

L. Mistakes in counting and calculations.

M. Presence of nucleated red cells, causing high white cell count.

N. Inaccurate pipettes or counting chambers.

O. Squeezing finger too much, thus diluting blood with tissue fluid.

PROGRAMMED QUESTIONS

Cover answers with a piece of paper.   Answers appear at end of questions.

(1) What is the dilution for a <u>normal</u> red blood cell count by hemocytometry?
(a) 50 times
(b) 250 times
(c) 200 times
(d) 20 times

(2) What is the volume of each W section on the hemocytometer slide?
(a) 0.1 mm^3
(b) 0.02 mm^3
(c) 0.4 mm^3
(d) 1 mm^3

(3) The red cell diluting fluid must be _____, with respect to the red cells.
(a) Hypotonic
(b) Isotonic
(c) Hypertonic
(d) None of the above

(4) Which of the following is a diluting fluid for the white cell count?
(a) Hayem's solution
(b) Sahli's solution
(c) 2% Acetic acid
(d) Gower's solution

(5) What should be done to the pipette as it is being filled with diluting fluid for a blood cell count?
   (a) Shaken
   (b) Rotated
   (c) Heated
   (d) Left alone

(6) What is one criterion for a properly filled counting chamber?
   (a) Fluid fills chamber entirely
   (b) Fluid fills chamber by capillary attraction only
   (c) Fluid does not run into groove
   (d) Both (a) and (c) are correct

(7) Under which power of the microscope do you count the white cells on the hemocytometer slide?
   (a) Scanning objective
   (b) Low dry objective
   (c) High dry objective
   (d) Oil immersion objective

(8) Each W and R section is subdivided into _____ small squares.
   (a) 80
   (b) 9
   (c) 400
   (d) 16

(9) What will increase a total white cell count?
   (a) Debris
   (b) Nucleated red cells
   (c) Air bubbles
   (d) Not discarding first 3 or 4 drops of diluting fluid from pipette before charging the counting chamber

(10) What is the combined normal white blood cell correction factor used in calculating the WBC count?
   (a) 250
   (b) 10,000
   (c) 25
   (d) 50

Answers

(1) c
(2) a
(3) b
(4) c
(5) b

(6) a
(7) b
(8) d
(9) b
(10) d

Erythrocyte Sedimentation Rate (ESR)

I. PRINCIPLES OF ERYTHROCYTE SEDIMENTATION RATE

The rate at which the red blood cells settle out from the plasma is the erythrocyte sedimentation rate. The sedimentation rate measures suspension stability of the erythrocytes. The cells settle because of their greater density as compared to the plasma. Essentially, sedimentation rate is an indication of amount and kind of plasma proteins in the plasma. The more viscous the plasma, the lower the sedimentation rate. Increasing the ratio of globulins to albumin results in a greater sedimentation rate.

Sedimentation rate tests are nonspecific, since rate is increased in all conditions in which there is tissue destruction and infection. In diseases, such as rheumatic fever, rheumatoid arthritis, cancer and tuberculosis, the sedimentation rate is increased. Sedimentation rate tests are useful guides in following the prognosis (course) and treatment of a disease. The return of an increased sedimentation rate to normal is a favorable indication that an inflammation is subsiding. The sedimentation rate is measured in millimeters per hour.

II. MODIFIED WESTERGREN SEDIMENTATION METHOD

This method is more reliable than others with blood having a rapid sedimentation rate because of the long column of blood that is used.

A. Materials

    1. Westergren Apparatus.—

        a. Westergren Pipette.—This is calibrated from 0–200 mm from top to bottom. The pipette holds 1.0 ml of blood.

        b. Westergren Rack.—This is a stand into which the pipette is placed.

    2. Blood.—Venipuncture anticoagulated blood is used which should not be more than 2 hr old. Otherwise, cells will swell and interfere with an accurate sedimentation rate.

The anticoagulant used for collection of blood for this method is either sodium citrate or EDTA, since these anticoagulants exert no effect on sedimentation rate. Heparin or oxalate may affect sedimentation rate by decreasing cell size.

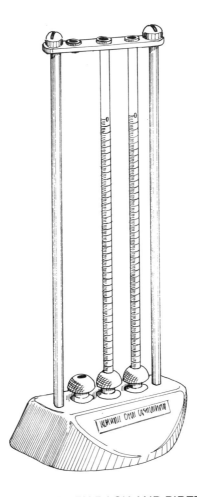

FIG. 6.1. WESTERGREN RACK AND PIPETTES

Since undiluted blood is too viscous for this test, the EDTA-anticoagulated blood is diluted with either 3.8% sodium citrate or 0.85% sodium chloride in a ratio of 1 part sodium citrate (or sodium chloride) to 4 parts blood. This ratio of salt to blood yields the proper dilution of the blood for the modified Westergren sedimentation test. (Some laboratories prefer to use 3.8% sodium citrate as the only anticoagulant in a ratio of 4 parts of blood to 1 of citrate. The diluted blood can then be set up directly in the Westergren tube with no further modification.)

B. Method

1. The blood and the 3.8% sodium citrate are thoroughly mixed to suspend the erythrocytes.

2. The Westergren pipette is filled with the diluted blood to slightly above the 0 mm mark. The blood is wiped from the outside and bottom of the pipette and then allowed to drain onto gauze exactly to the 0 mm mark (see Fig. 6.2).

3. **Insertion of Westergren Pipette into Westergren Rack.—**

    a. Place a piece of Parafilm on the rubber bumper at the base of the Westergren rack. The bottom of the Westergren pipette is firmly pressed against the bumper before removing the finger from the pipette.

b. The pipette is held firmly by the clip at the top of the rack in an exactly vertical position. If the pipette is not vertical, the cells will pile up on the side walls of the pipette, slide down and fall faster.

4. Set the timer for 1 hr. In exactly 1 hr, record as the sedimentation rate the number of millimeters the red cell meniscus has fallen.

5. **Average Fall and Index.**—These values can be calculated by allowing the sedimentation test to continue for 2 hr. Take the reading after first hour and divide the reading by 2; take reading after the second hour and divide the reading by 4. These values are the average falls per hour; add the 2 values together and record as the index. The reason for dividing first and second hour readings by 2 and 4, respectively, is that the red cell fall is in a geometric progression. The red cell fall each hour is not constant, since the packing effect of the red cells is greater the longer the time the red cells continue to fall.

Example: First hour reading, 10 mm; second hour reading, 25 mm.

$$
\text{Index} = \frac{\text{mm of red cell fall in first hour}}{2} + \frac{\text{mm of red cell fall in second hour}}{4}
$$

$$
= \frac{10}{2} + \frac{25}{4}
$$

$$
= 5 + 6.2
$$

$$
\text{Index} = 11.2
$$

Many laboratories do not report the index and consider the first hour reading as sufficient.

C. Normal Values for Westergren Sedimentation

Males	0–15 mm/hr
Females	0–20 mm/hr

Female sedimentation rate is higher than male sedimentation rate; it increases with age in both sexes.

D. Changes from Normal Sedimentation Rate of Erythrocytes

1. **Changes in Ratio of Erythrocytes to Plasma.**—

a. In anemia, where there is a decrease in red cells, sedimentation rate is increased, since a lowering in red cell number favors rouleaux formation. Rouleaux will fall faster than a single cell due to the combined weight of the cells.

(A) (B)

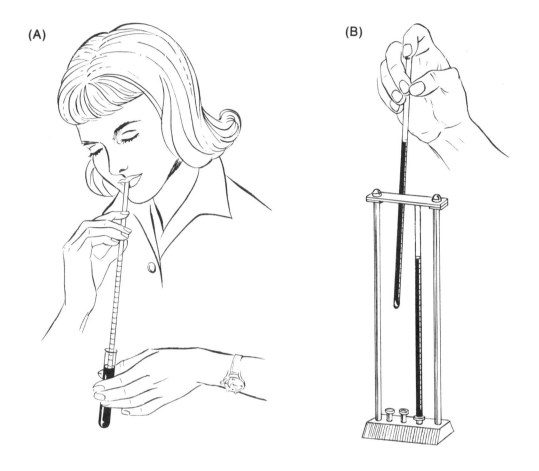

FIG. 6.2. (A) FILLING THE WESTERGREN PIPETTE. (B) PLACING IT IN THE WESTERGREN RACK

    b. In polycythemia, where there is an increase in red cells, sedimentation rate is decreased.

2. Change in Viscosity of the Plasma.—Extreme increase in plasma viscosity decreases sedimentation rate by preventing rouleaux formation. Decrease in plasma viscosity accelerates sedimentation rate.

    After the third month of pregnancy, the sedimentation rate increases due to decrease in plasma proteins.

    Lipids retard sedimentation rate, except cholesterol which accelerates it.

3. Specific Plasma Proteins' Effect on Sedimentation Rate.—

    a. Increased levels of fibrinogen increase rouleaux formation of red cells, increasing the sedimentation rate.
    b. Increase of globulins increases sedimentation rate.
    c. Elevated albumin levels decrease sedimentation rates.

    However, there is no absolute correlation between sedimentation rate and any plasma protein fraction.

4. Red Cell Factors' Effect on Sedimentation Rate.—

    a. Size of Red Cells.—Microcytes have a decreased sedimentation rate compared to macrocytes, while macrocytes sediment more rapidly than normocytes.

    b. Anisocytosis.—Irregularly sized cells do not allow for rouleaux formation, so sedimentation rate is decreased.

E. Stages in Sedimentation Rate

Three stages can be recognized.

1. **Initial Period of Aggregation.—**During the time rouleaux are forming, sedimentation is slow. This period is about 10 min.

2. **Period of Fast Settling.—**Rouleaux are of maximum size and settling rate is constant. This period lasts about 40 min.

3. **Final Period of Packing.—**This period continues for the remainder of the hour, or longer if sedimentation test is continued for longer than 1 hr.

III. CUTLER SEDIMENTATION METHOD

A. Materials

1. **Cutler Tube.—**This is graduated from 0–50 mm. The tube holds 1.0 ml of blood.

2. **Blood.—**Any anticoagulated venipuncture blood which is not more than 2 hr old can be used.

B. Method

1. Mix blood well to suspend the cells.
2. Fill Cutler tube to 0 mm mark with the blood.
3. Set the Cutler tube in a rack so it is exactly vertical.
4. At 5 min intervals, for 1 hr, read the number of millimeters the red cells have fallen. Record and plot results on a Cutler sedimentation rate graph.

IV. WINTROBE SEDIMENTATION METHOD

A. Materials

1. **Wintrobe Tube.—**This is graduated from 0–100 mm. The tube holds 1.0 ml of blood.

2. **Wintrobe Rack**

3. **Blood.—**Any anticoagulated venipuncture blood which is not more than 2 hr old can be used.

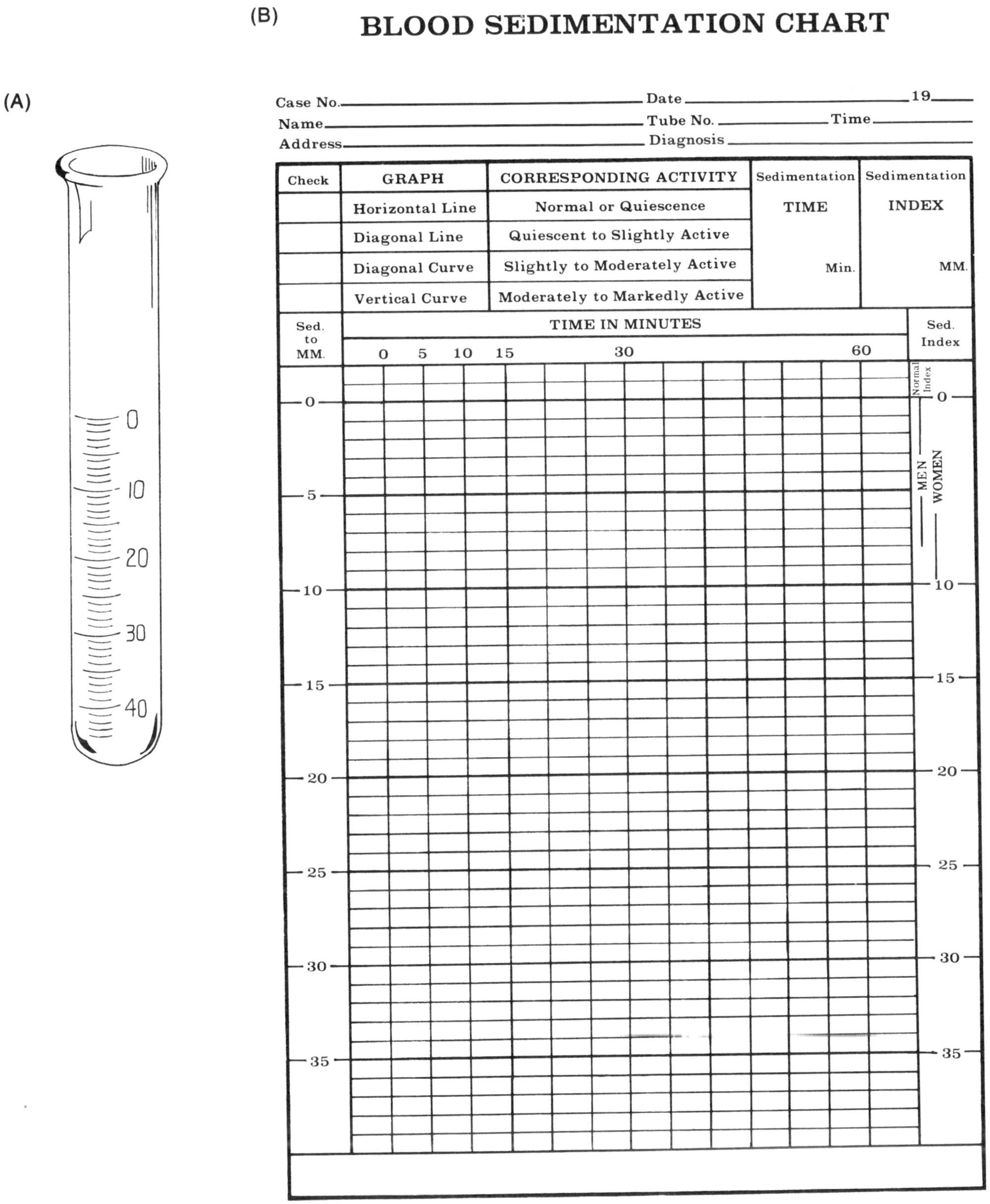
(A)
0
10
20
30
40
(B)
BLOOD SEDIMENTATION CHART
Case No.
Date
19
Name
Tube No.
Time
Address
Diagnosis
Check
GRAPH
CORRESPONDING ACTIVITY
Sedimentation TIME
Sedimentation INDEX
Horizontal Line
Normal or Quiescence
Diagonal Line
Quiescent to Slightly Active
Diagonal Curve
Slightly to Moderately Active
Vertical Curve
Moderately to Markedly Active
Min.
MM.
Sed. to MM.
TIME IN MINUTES
0 5 10 15 30 60
Sed. Index
Normal Index
MEN
WOMEN
0
5
10
15
20
25
30
35

FIG. 6.3. (A) CUTLER TUBE. (B) SEDIMENTATION RATE GRAPH

B. Method

1. Mix blood well to suspend the cells.
2. Fill the Wintrobe tube with blood by a Wintrobe pipette in the same manner as for Wintrobe macro-hematocrit (Fig. 4.3). Fill the tube exactly to the 0 mm mark.
3. Place the filled tube in the Wintrobe rack exactly vertical.
4. Set timer for 1 hr. After 1 hr read the left side of the Wintrobe tube and record as the sedimentation rate the distance the red cell meniscus has fallen.

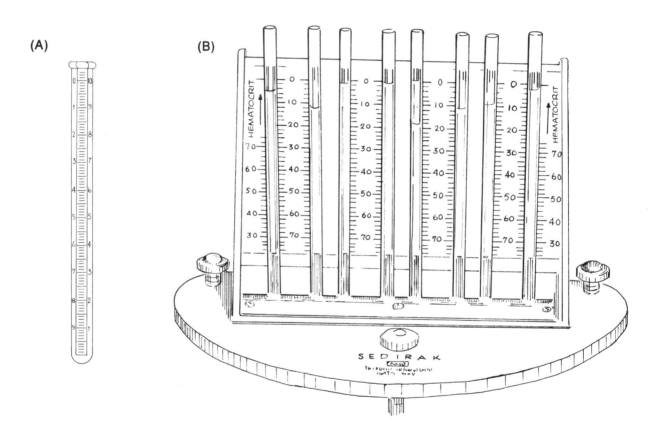

FIG. 6.4.   (A) WINTROBE SEDIMENTATION TUBE. (B) WINTROBE RACK

C. Normal Values for Wintrobe Sedimentation Rate

Male   0–9 mm/hr
Female   0–15 mm/hr

V. LANDAU MICRO-SEDIMENTATION METHOD

In this method fingertip or capillary blood is used. The micro method is used on children and when it is hard to obtain venous blood, as with arthritic patients. It is not considered to be as accurate as macro methods.

A. Materials

1. Landau pipette and stand.—The pipette resembles a red cell pipette. The stem of the pipette is graduated from 0–50 mm.
2. Suction device allows blood and anticoagulant to be drawn into pipette.
3. 5% Sodium citrate is the anticoagulant.
4. Blood.—Use fingertip blood or capillary blood.

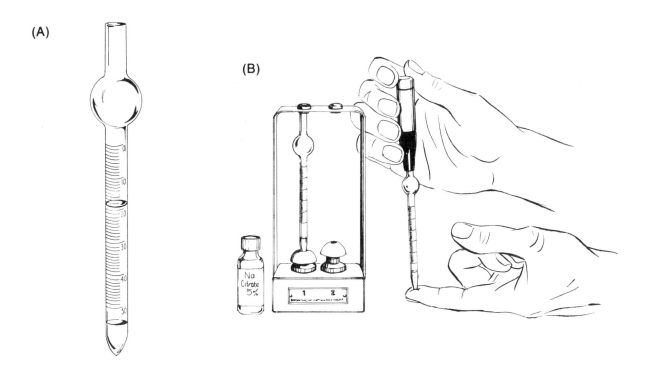

(A)

(B)

FIG. 6.5.   (A) LANDAU SEDIMENTATION PIPETTE. (B) SUCTION DEVICE AND RACK

B. Method

1. The Landau pipette is attached to the suction device.
2. 5% Sodium citrate is drawn up the stem of the pipette to the first line.
3. The fingertip puncture is made and a drop of blood is produced in the usual manner.
4. The tip of the pipette is put in the drop of blood and the blood is drawn up with the suction device until the mixture reaches the second line on the stem of the pipette. There should be no air bubbles in fluid column in the stem of the pipette.
5. The pipette is wiped clean of blood. By turning the knob of the suction device the mixture of 5% sodium citrate and blood is slowly drawn into the bulb of the pipette to be thoroughly mixed. The mixture is forced back and forth from bulb to stem several times to ensure mixing of the anticoagulant and the blood.
6. After the mixing, the mixture is forced back into the stem of the pipette. The upper level of the anticoagulated diluted mixed blood is set to the 0 mm mark. The lower level of the blood column should not touch the tip of the pipette.
7. Detach the suction device by placing finger over tip of pipette.

8. Place Landau pipette in the Landau rack in an exactly vertical position.
9. Set timer for 1 hr. After 1 hr record as the sedimentation rate how far the red cell meniscus has fallen.

C. Normal Values for Landau Micro–sedimentation Rate

Male   0–5 mm/hr
Female   0–8 mm/hr

VI. SOURCES OF ERROR IN THE SEDIMENTATION RATE

A. Unclean sedimentation tubes cause hemolysis, decrease sedimentation rate.
B. Excessive anticoagulant makes blood too viscous, decreases sedimentation rate.
C. Partially clotted blood will decrease sedimentation rate because plasma is too viscous.
D. Blood must be fresh, not more than 2 hr old after withdrawal. As blood stands some cells hemolyze; others swell, become more spherical, and do not form rouleaux. Decrease in rouleaux formation decreases sedimentation rate.
E. Failure to mix blood sufficiently before filling sedimentation tubes. Invert room temperature blood 10–12 times; invert refrigerated blood 10–20 times after blood returns to room temperature in order to suspend cells well.
F. Air bubbles in column of blood.
G. Inclined sedimentation tube.—Sedimentation pipettes and tubes must be placed exactly vertical in the sedimentation rack. Otherwise cells will pile up on the side walls of the tube and slide down faster to increase sedimentation rate.
H. Room temperature.—Room temperature must be constant. If room temperature is raised, sedimentation rate is higher.
I. Tube Diameter.—Tube diameter has to be standard at 2.5 mm; a smaller diameter decreases sedimentation rate.

Since this laboratory exercise is relatively short, students can repeat CBC procedure or other procedures at discretion of the instructor.

PROGRAMMED QUESTIONS

Cover answers with a piece of paper. Answers appear at end of questions.

(1) In which of the following would sedimentation rate be decreased?
(a) Pregnancy
(b) Rheumatoid arthritis
(c) Tuberculosis
(d) Polycythemia (vera or transitory)

(2) Which factor or factors influence sedimentation rate?
(a) Inclination of sedimentation tube
(b) Diameter of sedimentation tube
(c) Freshness of the blood
(d) All of the above

(3) Which of the following is not a sedimentation rate method?
(a) Landau
(b) Duke
(c) Westergren
(d) Wintrobe

(4) In the Westergren method, which anticoagulant is the one of choice?
(a) 3.8% Na citrate
(b) Heparin
(c) Oxalate
(d) Sodium chloride

(5) What is the normal sedimentation rate for a male by the Westergren method?
(a) 0–20 mm/hr
(b) 0–9 mm/hr
(c) 0–15 mm/hr
(d) 0–8 mm/hr

(6) Which sedimentation rate method uses only capillary blood?
(a) Drabkin's
(b) Landau
(c) Wintrobe
(d) Micro-capillary

(7) Which of the following would decrease rouleaux formation and thus decrease the sedimentation rate?
(a) Increase in albumin
(b) Air bubbles in column of blood
(c) Increase in temperature
(d) Increase in globulins

(8) The _____ side of the Wintrobe tube is read for sedimentation rate.
(a) Back
(b) Right
(c) Front
(d) Left

(9) Which mathematical expression describes the average fall of red cells during a sedimentation rate procedure?
(a) Logarithmic progression
(b) Geometric progression
(c) Arithmetric progression
(d) Linear progression

(10) What is the proper dilution of the blood with physiological saline solution in the modified Westergren sedimentation method?
(a) 2 Parts saline:4 parts blood
(b) 4 Parts saline:1 part blood
(c) 1 Part saline:4 parts blood
(d) Blood does not have to be diluted for this method

Answers

(1) d	(6) b
(2) d	(7) a
(3) b	(8) d
(4) a	(9) b
(5) c	(10) c

7

The Platelet Count

I. REES-ECKER DIRECT METHOD FOR PLATELET COUNT

A. Principles of the Direct Method

In the direct method, the number of platelets in diluted blood is counted in a specific volume on the hemocytometer slide. From this number, the platelets in undiluted blood are calculated and reported as number of platelets/mm³ of blood. Normal platelet values vary between 140,000–340,000/mm³ of blood, with 240,000–300,000/mm³ of blood as the average.

B. Materials

1. **Rees-Ecker Diluting Solution.**—The Rees-Ecker solution contains brilliant cresyl blue, sodium citrate and formaldehyde. This solution stains and preserves the platelets and red cells. It is always necessary to prefilter Rees-Ecker solution just before using in order to remove precipitated crystals of stain and other debris which may be mistaken for platelets.
2. **Red Cell Pipette**
3. **Hemocytometer Kit**
4. **Petri Dish Cover with Moist Paper Toweling**
5. **Blood.**—Capillary or freshly obtained venipuncture blood may be used. Blood must be fresh or platelets will disintegrate.

C. Method

1. Perform a fingertip puncture in the usual manner.
2. Draw blood up exactly to the 0.5 mark in the red cell pipette.
3. Fill pipette with Rees-Ecker solution to the 101 mark in the red cell pipette. Rotate pipette while filling.
4. Shake pipette by hand or on the mechanical shaker for 45 sec to mix the dilution.

5. Discard the first 3–4 drops from the pipette.
6. Charge either or both counting chambers with the diluted blood.[1]
7. Allow platelets to settle on counting chamber before counting by placing the charged hemocytometer slide under a Petri dish cover with moist paper toweling for 5–10 min. The placing of the hemocytometer slide under the Petri dish prevents evaporation of the fluid from the chambers.
8. Using the high power of the microscope, count the platelets in the 5 red cell sections or platelet sections. The platelets appear as tiny glistening objects about 1/10 the size of red cells. The platelets could be spherical, oval, rod-shaped or comma-shaped, either single or in groups. There should be about 3–8 platelets per platelet section.

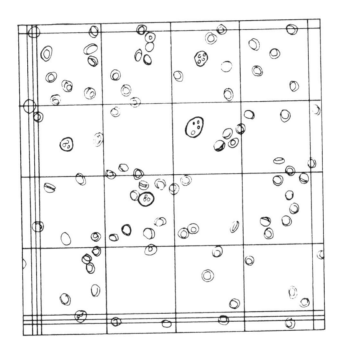

FIG. 7.1.   APPEARANCE OF PLATELETS IN A PLATELET SECTION.
PLATELETS ARE GLISTENING AND CIRCLED IN BLACK.

9. **Calculations.**—Add up the platelets counted in the 5 platelet sections and multiply the count by 10,000 or add 4 zeros.

Example: 30 platelets counted in the 5 platelet sections
30 × 10,000 = 300,000 platelets/mm³ of blood

10. To remove stain of the Rees-Ecker solution from the red cell pipette, rinse pipette in 70% alcohol and allow pipette to soak for a few hours in the 70% alcohol.

---

[1]It is possible to charge the upper chamber with white cells for a total white cell count and the lower chamber with the Rees-Ecker diluted blood. In this way both the platelets and red cells may be counted, since the same dilutions are made for both.

D. Difficulties in Enumeration of Platelets

1. Small size of platelets as seen under high dry objective.
2. Debris can be mistaken for platelets.
3. Uneven distribution of platelets among the 5 platelet sections.
4. Oil immersion lens cannot be used to observe platelets in the hemocytometer slide.

E. Errors in Platelet Count

1. **Decreased Platelet Count.—**

    a. **Squeezing Finger.—**This decreases platelet count by causing disintegration and agglutination of platelets.

    b. **Dirty Glassware.—**Platelets stick to the dirt.

2. **Increased Platelet Count.—**Debris and precipitated stain in diluting fluid can be mistaken for platelets.

F. Preparation of Rees–Ecker Solution

Brilliant cresyl blue	0.1 g
Sodium citrate	3.8 g
40% Formaldehyde	0.2 ml
Distilled water to	100 ml

Filter before use.

II. FONIO INDIRECT METHOD FOR PLATELET COUNT

A. Principles of the Indirect Method

In the indirect method, the ratio of platelets to red cells is estimated by counting the platelets on the blood smear and by performing a red cell count on the hemocytometer.

B. Materials

1. 14% Magnesium sulfate ($MgSO_4$)—diluting fluid
2. Glass slides for blood smear
3. Red cell pipette
4. Hemocytometer kit, Hayem's solution
5. Wright's stain or Hema-tek

C. Method

1. Disinfect finger with 70% alcohol.
2. Then place a drop of 14% $MgSO_4$ solution on the ball of the finger; make a fingertip puncture through the $MgSO_4$ solution. This dilutes the blood and prevents clumping and disintegration of the platelets.
3. Gently squeeze the finger so blood flows out and mixes with the $MgSO_4$ solution.
4. Make 2 blood smears.
5. Wipe fingertip, produce another drop of blood, collect blood with red cell pipette for a red cell count. Perform a red cell count on the hemocytometer. Calculate results as RBC/mm^3 of blood.
6. Stain the blood smear with Wright's stain manually or by Hema-tek.
7. On the stained blood smear count 1000 red cells under oil immersion lens and record the number of platelets seen during the count. To facilitate the red cell count and platelet count so as to count these structures only once, narrow the microscopic fields by using a window. Insert window onto top of the eyepiece. To make a window, use an index card; cut out a circle of same diameter as eyepiece. Cut a window in center of the circle; insert window on top of eyepiece.

8. **Calculations.—**

$$\text{platelet count} = \frac{\text{(number of platelets counted on the blood smear)}}{\text{(number of red cells counted on the blood smear)}} \times \begin{array}{c} \text{red cell count on} \\ \text{hemocytometer} \end{array}$$

Example: RBC count on hemocytometer = $5{,}000{,}000/mm^3$ of blood
RBC counted on blood smear = 1000
Platelets counted on blood smear = 50

$$\text{platelet count} = \frac{50}{1000} \times 5{,}000{,}000 = 250{,}000, \text{platelets}/mm^3 \text{ of blood}$$

The indirect method gives higher values than the direct method and is less accurate. Since this exercise is relatively short, students can repeat CBC procedure or other procedures at the discretion of the instructor.

D. Preparation of 14% Magnesium Sulfate

Magnesium sulfate	14 g
Distilled water to	100 ml

PROGRAMMED QUESTIONS

Cover answers with a piece of paper.   Answers appear at end of questions.

(1) In the Rees-Ecker method for the plate-let count, which sections of the hemocy-tometer slide are used?
(a) 4 W sections
(b) All W sections
(c) 5 R sections
(d) All R sections

(2) After you charge the hemocytometer slide in the Rees-Ecker method for platelet count, why must you wait 5–10 min before making the count?
(a) During this time platelets are settling on the counting chamber's platform
(b) During this time there is no evapora-tion of fluids from the counting chamber
(c) During this time you are performing the red cell count
(d) During this time the brilliant cresyl blue is precipitating out of solution

(3) What is one difficulty encountered in counting platelets by the Rees-Ecker method?
(a) Small sized platelets as viewed under high dry objective
(b) Debris mistakenly recognized as platelets
(c) No even distribution of platelets
(d) All of the above

(4) In the Rees-Ecker method, to obtain platelets/mm^3 of blood, multiply the number of platelets by _____.
(a) 50
(b) 10,000
(c) 250
(d) 1000

(5) Which pipette and what ratio of blood to diluting fluid are used in performing a normal platelet count by the Rees-Ecker method?
(a) Red cell pipette, 0.5:101
(b) Red cell pipette, 0.5:11
(c) White cell pipette, 0.5:101
(d) White cell pipette, 0.5:11

(6) What is the name of the method for the indirect platelet count?
(a) Wintrobe
(b) Rees-Ecker
(c) Lee-White
(d) None of the above

(7) What is the function of the 14% $MgSO_4$ placed on the ball of the finger in the indirect platelet count?
(a) Prevent precipitation of the brilliant cresyl blue
(b) Prevent clumping and disintegra-tion of platelets
(c) Clear the Wright's stain of debris
(d) Cause hemolysis of the red cells

(8) What must be counted in addition to platelets in the indirect method for counting of platelets?
(a) Red cells on hemocytometer slide
(b) White cells on blood smear
(c) 1000 Red cells on blood smear
(d) Both (a) and (c)

(9) Platelets are about _____ size of red cells.
   (a) 0.1
   (b) 0.5
   (c) 2 Times
   (d) None of the above

(10) In order to count platelets, blood must be _____.
   (a) Anticoagulated
   (b) Refrigerated
   (c) Fresh
   (d) Well-suspended

Answers

(1) c	(6) d
(2) a	(7) b
(3) d	(8) d
(4) b	(9) a
(5) a	(10) c

8

The Reticulocyte Count

I. PRINCIPLES OF THE RETICULOCYTE COUNT

The reticulocytes are normally about 1% of the red cells in the peripheral blood (50,000–60,000/mm^3 of blood). The reticulocyte count is significant since it tells whether the bone marrow is producing red cells at a proper rate, thus indicating the conditions in the bone marrow. Decreased red cell production in the bone marrow (hypoplastic or aplastic) leads to a drop in reticulocyte count in the peripheral blood (reticulocytopenia). Increased red cell production in the bone marrow (hyperplastic) leads to a rise in the reticulocytes in the peripheral blood (reticulocytosis). Reticulocytosis is found in conditions of hereditary spherocytosis, sickle cell anemia, thalassemia, various hemolytic anemias and acute hemorrhage. Reticulocytopenia is found in conditions of aplastic anemia and pernicious anemia. ↓Retic   mean low

The reticulocytes are slightly larger than erythrocytes, but in Wright's stained blood smears they cannot be distinguished from erythrocytes since both stain the same. The reticulocytes contain a net-like reticulum in their cytoplasm which is the remains of the RNA. This reticulum can be visualized if blood is fresh and the cells are stained by a supravital stain. A supravital stain is one that stains the cells in the living condition, not after a blood smear is made. The supravital stains must be prefiltered just before use, as the particles of stain precipitate out of solution and can be mistaken for the net-like reticulum as they precipitate out upon the cells of the smear. Thus particles of stain precipitating on erythrocytes would make them appear like reticulocytes (see Fig. 8.1).

II. MATERIALS

A. Supravital Stains (Prefilter Before Use)

1% Brilliant cresyl blue in 0.85% NaCl
1% New methylene blue N in 0.85% NaCl
1% Brilliant cresyl blue in methyl alcohol

To each solution add 3.8 g of sodium citrate per 100 ml of solution to act as an anticoagulant.

B. Heparinized capillary tubes, toothpick

C. Glass slides

D. Blood.—Fingertip blood or fresh EDTA-anticoagulated venipuncture blood can be used.

III. METHOD

The reticulocyte count is made by the dry method.

A. Make a fingertip puncture in the usual manner.
B. Fill 1 heparinized capillary tube 3/4 full of blood.
C. Fill a second capillary tube with prefiltered supravital stain.
D. Mix blood and stain together on a slide with a toothpick.
E. Take up stained blood in a third capillary tube.
F. Allow cells to accept the stain for 10 min or longer.
G. Then tap out 1 or 2 drops of stained blood from capillary tube at one end of 2 slides and make 2 blood smears. Allow to dry.
H. Dry the supravitally stained smear and observe under the oil immersion lens. Use a window in the eyepiece to decrease size of the microscopic field to facilitate counting (see Exercise 7).
I. On the thin end of the smear where the red cells are uniformly distributed, count 1000 red cells (erythrocytes and reticulocytes) while also recording the number of reticulocytes observed.
J. Calculate the percentage of reticulocytes according to the formula:

$$\% \text{ reticulocytes} = \frac{(\text{number of reticulocytes counted})}{(1000 \text{ red cells}\,[\text{erythrocytes} + \text{reticulocytes}]\text{ counted})} \times 100$$

Example: Number of reticulocytes counted while counting 1000 red cells = 10

$$\% \text{ reticulocytes} = \frac{10}{1000} \times 100$$
$$= 1\%$$

K. Report the method and result.

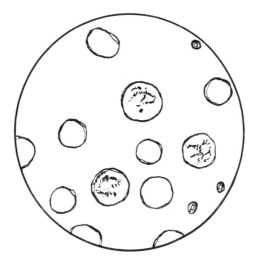

FIG. 8.1.   RETICULOCYTES STAINED BY SUPRAVITAL STAIN.
THE CYTOPLASM OF THE CELL IS STAINED LIGHT GREEN-BLUE
AND THE RETICULUM DEEP BLUE.

Since this exercise is extremely short, students can repeat elements of other laboratory sections at the discretion and direction of the instructor.

PROGRAMMED QUESTIONS

Cover answers with a piece of paper.   Answers appear at end of questions.

(1) Which supravital stain is used for reticulocytes?
(a) Ferricyanide
(b) Methyl alcohol
(c) Brilliant cresyl blue
(d) Eosin

(2) Reticulocytes are slightly _____ than erythrocytes and contain a reticulum of _____.
(a) Larger, DNA
(b) Larger, RNA
(c) Smaller, RNA
(d) Smaller, DNA

(3) A reticulocytopenia is a reflection of _____.
(a) Increased production of neutrophils in the bone marrow
(b) Increased production of red cells in the bone marrow
(c) Decreased production of platelets in the bone marrow
(d) Decreased production of red cells in the bone marrow

(4) In performance of the reticulocyte count by the "dry" method, how many red cells are counted while counting the reticulocytes?
(a) 1000
(b) 990
(c) 10,000
(d) 10

(5) What is the normal reticulocyte count?
(a) 5000–10,000/mm^3 of blood
(b) 42%
(c) 1–2%
(d) 14.5 g/100 ml of blood

(6) In which condition is a reticulocytosis found?
(a) Sickle cell anemia
(b) Aplastic anemia
(c) Pernicious anemia
(d) None of the above

(7) Why must the supravital stain be prefiltered?
(a) Particles of stain precipitating on reticulocytes make them appear as erythrocytes
(b) Particles of stain precipitating on reticulocytes make reticulocytes appear as eosinophils
(c) Particles of stain precipitating appear as reticulocytes
(d) Particles of stain precipitating on erythrocytes make them appear as reticulocytes

Answers

(1) c   (5) c
(2) b   (6) a
(3) d   (7) d
(4) a

9

Mean Corpuscular Values and Erythrocyte Indexes

The mean corpuscular values and erythrocyte indexes are calculated from the red cell count, hemoglobin, and hematocrit estimations. These primary values must be accurate or the secondary, calculated values will not be correct.

I. MEAN CORPUSCULAR VALUES

There are three mean corpuscular values.

A. Significance of Mean Corpuscular Values

These values are concerned with the volume of the average erythrocyte (size) and the amount of hemoglobin in the average erythrocyte and are useful in the classification of anemias.

B. Mean Corpuscular Volume (MCV)

1. **Definition.**—Volume of the average erythrocyte (size). MCV indicates whether red cells are microcytic, normocytic or macrocytic.

2. **Normal Values.**—80–90 cubic microns (μ^3)

3. **Calculation.**—

$$MCV = \frac{\text{hematocrit as percentage}}{\text{RBC in millions}} \times 10$$

Based on findings of:

Hematocrit = 40%
Hb = 14 g/100 ml blood
RBC count = 5,000,000/mm^3 of blood

$$\text{Example:}\quad \text{MCV} = \frac{40}{5.0} \times 10 = 80\,\mu^3$$

C. Mean Corpuscular Hemoglobin (MCH)

1. **Definition.**—Weight of hemoglobin in the average erythrocyte. A low MCH can be found in either microcytic or normocytic red cells. An increase of MCH is found in macrocyte cells.

2. **Normal Values.**—27–32 micromicrograms $(\mu\mu\mathrm{g})$

3. **Calculation.**—

$$\text{MCH} = \frac{\text{Hb in grams}}{\text{RBC in millions}} \times 10$$

$$\text{Example:}\quad \text{MCH} = \frac{14}{5.0} \times 10$$
$$= 28\,\mu\mu\mathrm{g}$$

D. Mean Corpuscular Hemoglobin Concentration (MCHC)

1. **Definition.**—The grams of hemoglobin per milliliter of packed red cells or hematocrit. The value is expressed as percentage, so it is multiplied by 100; thus the mean corpuscular hemoglobin concentration is the percentage of hemoglobin in the hematocrit or packed cell volume. The MCHC indicates whether the cells are normochromic or hypochromic.

2. **Normal Values.**—33–38%

3. **Calculation.**—

$$\text{MCHC} = \frac{\text{Hb in grams}}{\text{hematocrit}} \times 100$$

$$\text{Example:}\quad \text{MCHC} = \frac{14}{40} \times 100$$
$$= 0.35 \times 100$$
$$= 35\%$$

All the above values are decreased in iron deficiency anemia. The first two values are increased during pernicious anemia. The last value cannot be increased above normal values because hemoglobin saturation of a cell is limited by the size of the erythrocyte. The larger the erythrocyte, the more hemoglobin it can hold. This amount of hemoglobin is normal for this size cell, but is greater than that for a normal-sized erythrocyte.

II. ERYTHROCYTE INDEXES

A. Types of Erythrocyte Indexes and Significance of the Indexes

There are three erythrocyte indexes: volume index (VI), saturation index (SI) and color index (CI). Color index is most commonly used and it should be calculated every time a red cell count and hemoglobin estimation are performed in order to check on the accuracy of the red cell count and hemoglobin estimation.

B. Standard Values

The erythrocyte indexes are a comparison of the patient's red cell count, hemoglobin concentration and hematocrit to standard values for these parameters. Volume index is a relationship of hematocrit to red cell count. Saturation index is a relationship of hemoglobin to hematocrit. Color index is a relationship of hemoglobin to red cell count.

The standard values are:

RBC count	5,000,000/mm^3 of blood
Hemoglobin	14.5 g/100 ml blood or 100% Hb
Hematocrit	42%

C. Color Index

Since color index is most commonly used, the following discussion involves this index mainly.

   1.   Calculation.—

   a. Long Method.—

$$\text{color index (CI)} = \frac{\dfrac{\text{patient's Hb}}{\text{standard Hb}}}{\dfrac{\text{patient's RBC count}}{\text{standard RBC count}}}$$

Hb values can be expressed as either g/100 ml blood or %Hb.

b. **Short Method.—**

$$CI = \frac{Hb \text{ in } \%}{(\text{first 2 digits in RBC count}) \times 2}$$

Example: *Given Values*
Hb   76%
RBC count   4,000,000/mm³ of blood

$$CI = \frac{76}{40 \times 2} = 0.95$$

2. **Normal Values.—**If patient's values are close to standard values, then all erythrocyte indexes should be close to 1.0 (0.9–1.1). Thus a value of 0.95 is normal as the patient's values come close to the standard values.

All three erythrocyte indexes are decreased in iron deficiency anemia. Volume and color indexes are increased during pernicious anemia. This is because erythrocytes are larger and hold more hemoglobin.

3. **Performance of the Color Index Test.—**The color index is a rough indication of how much hemoglobin is in the red cells. It is a useful guide to the technician, as it will point out gross errors between hemoglobin and red cell estimations and the appearance of the red cells on stained red cell examination. The color index tells you what the color of the red cells should be in the blood smear.

a. **Normochromic State.—**If the color index is about 1.0 on red cell examination, the red cells should be normally full of hemoglobin, with a small light central area. This is the normochromic state.

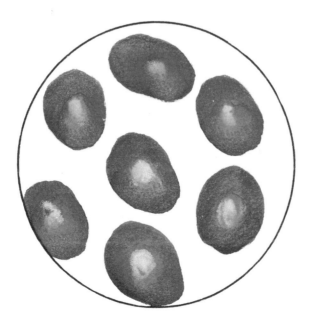

FIG. 9.1. RED CELLS WITH NORMAL AMOUNT OF HEMOGLOBIN: CI = 1.0 (SEE COLOR ATLAS)

b. **Hypochromic State.—**

(1) *Moderate.*—If the color index is about 0.5 on red cell examination, the red cells should be only 1/2 full of hemoglobin, with a larger light central area.

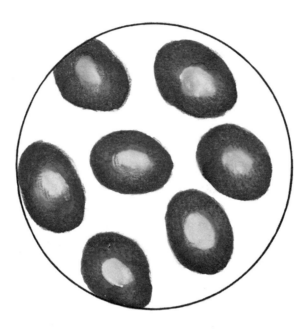

FIG. 9.2. RED CELLS WITH ONE-HALF THE NORMAL
AMOUNT OF HEMOGLOBIN: CI = 0.5 (SEE COLOR ATLAS)

(2) *Extreme.*—If the color index is about 0.1 on red cell examination, the red cells should be 0.1 full of hemoglobin, have a very large light central area and a thin peripheral red area. This is the hypochromic state.

c. **Hyperchromic State.—**Theoretically this state is physiologically impossible, as amount of hemoglobin depends on size of cell, and the hemoglobin usually saturates the cell to its full extent and not any more.

d. **Performing the Color Index Test.—**In performing a color index evaluation, the following procedure is used.
(1) Performance of hemoglobin estimation
(2) Red cell count
(3) Calculation of the color index
(4) From the calculation of color index, attempt to predict how the red cells should appear in the stained blood smear.
(5) Examination of the stained red cells on the blood smear to verify the prediction. If you worked accurately in performing hemoglobin and red cell estimation, there should be no discrepancy between what the red cells should look like and what they actually do look like on examination. If the red cells do not look like what you predicted them to be, there is a mistake in the red cell count or hemoglobin estimation or both and these tests should be repeated.

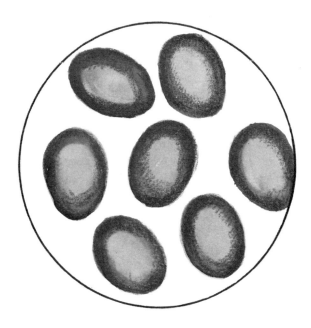

FIG. 9.3. RED CELLS CONTAINING ONE-TENTH THE NORMAL
AMOUNT OF HEMOGLOBIN: CI = 0.1 (SEE COLOR ATLAS)

III. DIFFERENCE BETWEEN MEAN CORPUSCULAR VALUES AND ERYTHROCYTE INDEXES

Mean corpuscular values are actual values of the patient's blood. The erythrocyte indexes are comparative values which compare patient's blood to the standard values. However, these values by themselves are not sufficient, but should be accompanied by a stained red cell examination on the blood smear. The stained red cell examination when properly performed offers valuable qualitative information concerning the size of the red cell and the hemoglobin content of the red cell.

IV. CORRELATION OF RED CELL COUNT AND HEMOGLOBIN VALUE

This relationship is direct, that is, as one of these values goes up or down the other usually does likewise. Thus you can make a rough approximate red cell estimation by multiplying the hemoglobin in percent by 5 and adding the proper number of zeros to give the red cell count in millions.

Example: Hb 11.6 g/100 ml blood is equivalent to 80%
5 stands for 5,000,000 RBC/mm³ of blood

$$80 \times 5 = 400 + 0000$$
$$= 4,000,000 \text{ RBC/mm}^3 \text{ of blood}$$

PROGRAMMED QUESTIONS

Cover answers with a piece of paper.   Answers appear at end of questions.

(1) If the erythrocyte has a MCV of 96 μ^3 a condition of _____ exists.
  (a) Macrocytosis
  (b) Hypochromia
  (c) Microcytosis
  (d) Normochromia

(2) The   MCHC   is   determined   by _____.
  (a) Multiplying hematocrit by 100 and dividing by RBC in millions
  (b) Dividing Hb in g by hematocrit and multiplying by 2
  (c) Dividing Hb in g by hematocrit
  (d) Dividing Hb in g by hematocrit and multiplying by 100

(3) The MCH is _____.
  (a) Volume of the average erythrocyte
  (b) Weight of hemoglobin in the average erythrocyte
  (c) Ratio of patient's hemoglobin to patient's red cell count
  (d) Percentage of hemoglobin in the packed red cell volume

(4) What is the main difference between mean corpuscular values and erythrocyte indexes?
  (a) Mean corpuscular values are comparative values; erythrocyte indexes are actual values
  (b) Mean corpuscular values are calculated values; erythrocyte indexes are comparative values
  (c) Mean corpuscular values are actual values; erythrocyte indexes are comparative values
  (d) There is no difference between mean corpuscular values and erythrocyte indexes

(5) To calculate a color index one must know the patient's and standard values for _____.
  (a) Hemoglobin and hematocrit
  (b) Hemoglobin and red cell count
  (c) Hematocrit and red cell count
  (d) Red cell count and white cell count

(6) What is considered to be the normal range for all erythrocyte indexes?
  (a) 0.9–1.1
  (b) 1.0–2.1
  (c) 1.0–1.5
  (d) 0.5–0.9

(7) What state of chromia would exist if the CI = 0.3?
  (a) Hyperchromia
  (b) Hypochromia
  (c) Normochromia
  (d) There is no chromic state for a CI = 0.3

(8) What is the CI if the patient has a red cell count of 4,500,000/mm^3 of blood and hemoglobin of 10.5 g/100 ml blood or 72%?
  (a) 0.90
  (b) 0.83
  (c) 1.02
  (d) 0.78

(9) Which of the following will give a rough approximation of a red cell count?
(a) Hb in % × 5 + 0000
(b) Hb in % × 5 × 0000
(c) Hb in g × 5 + 0000
(d) Hb in g + 5 × 0000

(10) What is the MCH if hematocrit is 45%, Hb 13.9 g/100 ml blood, and red cell count is 5,350,000/mm^3 of blood?
(a) 26%
(b) 26 μ^3
(c) 26 $\mu\mu$g
(d) None of the above

Answers

(1) a	(6) a
(2) d	(7) b
(3) b	(8) d
(4) c	(9) a
(5) b	(10) c

Automatic Cell Counting

The instrument most frequently used (though not the only one available) in the clinical laboratory for automatic cell counting is the Coulter Counter. The Model F Coulter Counter can perform the red cell count, the white cell count, and platelet counts, and, with the attached computers, also hematocrit and MCV. The Model S Coulter Counter, in addition, can estimate hemoglobin concentration, MCH and MCHC. The Model S is completely automatic from the time the undiluted sample is placed into the instrument until the results are printed out on a card. In using the Model F, dilution of the blood samples and the reporting of results are manual. This instrument is also an excellent teaching device as it demonstrates fundamental principles of cell counting.

I. GENERAL PRINCIPLES OF OPERATION

The Coulter Counter is basically a mercury manometer type syphon which creates a vacuum. The vacuum causes a flow of fluid through an opening or aperture in the aperture tube. If the fluid in the sample beaker is an electrolyte, an electric current or aperture current could pass between the electrodes inside and outside of the aperture tube. However, if cells or particles suspended in the electrolyte are poor conductors of electricity or cannot conduct electricity, then as the cells pass through the aperture, the current between the 2 electrodes momentarily decreases, producing a voltage drop for each cell. The magnitude or size of the voltage drop is proportional to size or volume of each cell. The voltage drops are fed into a complex electric circuit, which can discriminate between different amounts of voltage drops. The electric circuit then generates counting pulses for those cells that are larger than a certain size or above a threshold level, thus counting the number of cells.

In summary, the Coulter Counter uses the cells to interrupt a flow of electric current between 2 electrodes and counts the voltage drops produced by cells of threshold size or larger.

The mercury manometer between the start and stop electrodes is a horizontal U-shaped tube, which holds a 0.5 ml volume. As the mercury is being drawn through the manometer from start to stop electrode, 0.5 ml of diluted blood sample is drawn through the aperture and cells of threshold size or larger will be counted.

II. TYPE OF BLOOD TO USE

Capillary, fingertip blood, or venipuncture EDTA or heparinized blood can be used, but not oxalated blood. The oxalated blood with saponin (see following) causes a rapid deterioriation of the white cells.

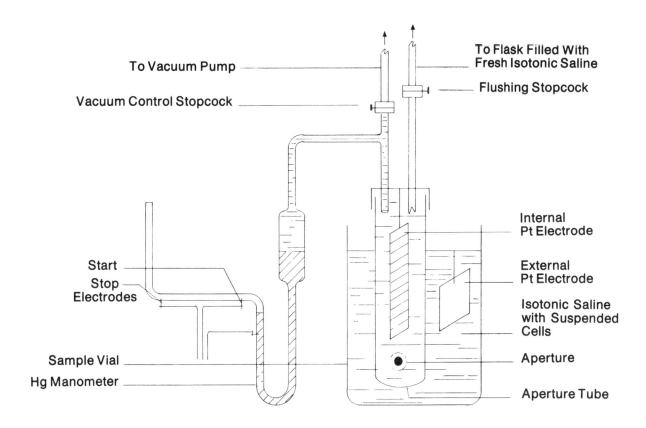

To Vacuum Pump

Vacuum Control Stopcock

To Flask Filled With
Fresh Isotonic Saline

Flushing Stopcock

Start
Stop
Electrodes

Internal
Pt Electrode

External
Pt Electrode

Isotonic Saline
with Suspended
Cells

Sample Vial

Aperture

Hg Manometer

Aperture Tube

FIG. 10.1.   PRINCIPLE OF THE COULTER COUNTER

III. DILUTION OF THE BLOOD CELLS

A. White Blood Cells

For the white cell count, the blood is diluted 1:500 with Isoton, a highly filtered saline solution. The dilution is best performed with an automatic dilutor (see Fig. 10.2). Into a disposable, clean 15 ml snap-cap plastic vial, add 0.02 ml of well-mixed blood to 10 ml of Isoton. Invert the diluted sample several times to uniformly suspend the cells, but avoid foaming. The red cells and platelets in the blood are lysed with 3 drops of 1% saponin solution (commercial name Zaponin, Zapiton or Zapisoton) so that they will not be counted with the white cells. On addition of saponin the cloudy red cell suspension becomes clear. If the red cells are to be counted, saponin is not added until red cell dilution is made. The Isoton and Zaponin have expiration dates which should be adhered to strictly.

B. Red Blood Cells

For the red cell count, the blood is diluted 1:50,000 with Isoton. Into a second vial, add 0.1 ml of diluted blood from the white cell suspension to 10 ml of Isoton. This makes a 1:100 dilution, but the final red cell dilution from the blood is 1:50,000 (500 × 100 = 50,000). The white cells and platelets are counted with the red cells, but their number, being small, adds an insignificant error to the red cell count.

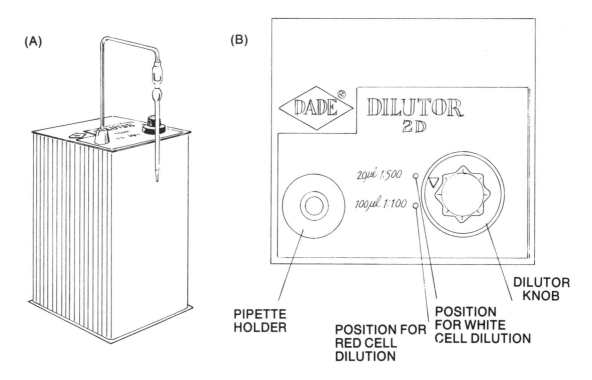

FIG. 10.2.   (A) AUTOMATIC DILUTOR
(B) POSITIONS OF SWITCH FOR WHITE AND RED CELL DILUTIONS

IV. PARTS OF THE MODEL F COULTER COUNTER

A. Digital Readout Assembly

The digital readout consists of 5 glow tubes. The white cell count is read directly off the glow tubes, from tubes 2 through 5 (from left to right) and reported as WBC/mm^3 of blood. The red cell count cannot be read directly off the glow tubes. The count must be multiplied by 100 to obtain RBC/mm^3 of blood. This is necessary due to the 1:100 dilution when the red cell dilution was made from the diluted blood of the white cell dilution.

B. Dual Monitor

The monitors are the oscilloscope and the debris monitor. They should be watched for irregularities during the count.

1.   **Oscilloscope.**—The oscilloscope displays as vertical lines or spikes the magnitude of the voltage drop for each individual cell passing through the aperture. The height of each spike is proportional to the voltage drop produced by the size of the cell passing through the aperture. This then checks on the size of the cells.

If the voltage drops generated for cells are all of the same size, the oscilloscope pattern should be practically uniform in height. If the oscilloscope displays irregularities in spike pattern, the cell suspension contains debris and irregular-sized cells. This then checks on the size distribution of the cells.

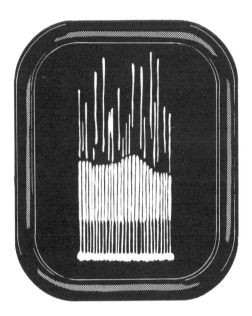

FIG. 10.3.   NORMAL OSCILLOSCOPE PATTERN

2.   **Debris Monitor.**—The debris monitor is an optical micro-projection system which allows for visual inspection of the aperture. The system consists of a projection lamp, mirror and objective lens. The mirror reflects the light of the projection lamp onto the aperture. The objective lens focuses the aperture onto the debris monitor. The monitor checks if the aperture is clear of debris or blocked with debris. If debris blocks the aperture, it is brushed away with a soft brush (see Fig. 10.4).

C. Sensitivity Controls

The magnitude of the voltage drops generated is directly proportional to the aperture current and the system's amplification. The aperture current is the electric current across the aperture between the 2 electrodes.

The sensitivity control values are set when the counter is first set up and calibrated. These values are determined for each specific instrument and, once established, are not changed as long as the same kind of particles is being counted.

1.   **Attenuation Control.**—The attenuation control adjusts the system's overall sensitivity with regard to electronic amplification. This control makes the system louder or softer, as a volume control works on a radio.

2.   **Aperture Current Control.**—The aperture current control controls the amount of aperture current between the 2 electrodes. Increasing the aperture current produces a larger voltage drop and larger spike height on the oscilloscope for a given size of cell. Decreasing aperture current will decrease the spike height for a given size of cell.

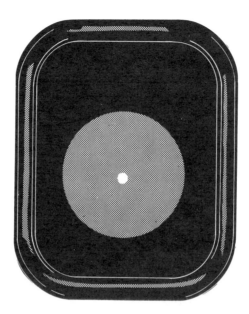

FIG. 10.4.   DEBRIS MONITOR

3. **Threshold or Discriminator Dial.**—The threshold dial controls the level of the size of cells above which cells will be counted. Thus all cells' causing a voltage drop of this particular size or larger in the 0.5 ml of fluid drawn through the aperture will be counted. Particles below the threshold level will not be counted. In routine cell counting the threshold control is at a low setting so as to count the smallest cells that might be encountered in the sample.

D. On-off Power Switch

Instrument should be turned on at least 10 min before operating to warm up (as the Model F contains vacuum tubes) and to give time for a vacuum to build up in the system.

E. Sample Stand Assembly

1. **Sample Platform.**—The sample platform is a spring-activated platform on which the sample vial is placed.

2. **Aperture Tube.**—The aperture tube contains the aperture through which cells in the diluted blood pass. The aperture size for white and red cells is 100 μ. For platelets, the aperture tube has an aperture of 75 μ. This tube is stored behind the sample stand assembly. The aperture tube should be positioned so that the aperture is close to the bottom and left side of the sample vial without the aperture tube's touching the sample vial. This position of the aperture tube ensures sharp projection of aperture in the debris monitor.

3. **Platinum Electrodes.—**

   a. Internal electrode inside the aperture tube
   b. External electrode outside the aperture tube, immersed in the diluted sample. Keep the electrode above and behind the aperture so as not to block the light shining on the aperture. If light is blocked, aperture cannot be viewed in the debris monitor.

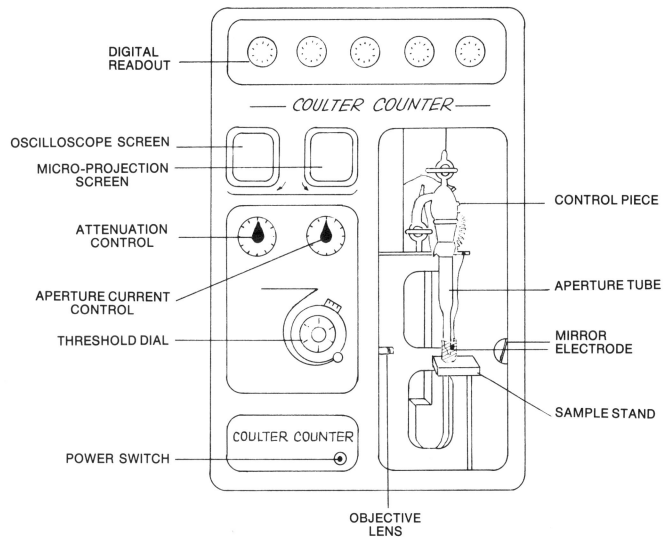

FIG. 10.5.   FRONT VIEW MODEL F COULTER COUNTER

4. **Mercury Manometer.—**The mercury manometer, located behind the sample platform, is a horizontal U-shaped tube, 0.5 ml in volume from start to stop electrode. The mercury manometer controls the exact amount of diluted sample to be syphoned from the sample vial. When the mercury contacts the stop electrode, the syphoning action stops and the instrument stops counting. The time for 0.5 ml of mercury to go from start to stop electrode is 13–15 sec. During this time, cells of threshold size or larger present in the 0.5 ml diluted sample drawn through the aperture are counted. This is about 50,000 red cells with a 1:50,000 dilution.

5. **Control Piece.**—The control piece is the base for mounting the aperture tube by a spring. The control piece contains 2 stopcocks which control the syphoning action of the manometer.

   a. **Vacuum Control Stopcock.**—Opening this stopcock (in vertical position) creates a negative pressure or vacuum in the manometer as the manometer is connected to a vacuum pump. The mercury is drawn below the start electrode and the counter resets to 0. When the stopcock is closed (in horizontal position) the mercury in the unbalanced manometer rises in the open leg of the manometer. This creates the syphoning action. When the mercury reaches the start electrode the counter starts to count the cells as 0.5 ml of diluted sample is drawn through the aperture. When 0.5 ml of mercury reaches the stop electrode, the count is finished. The mercury continues to rise in the manometer until equilibrium is reached.

   b. **Flushing Stopcock.**—This stopcock flushes out the aperture tube with fresh Isoton from an auxillary flask at the side of the counter. The aperture tube is flushed every time you change from one cell type to another. It is not necessary to flush the aperture tube between different samples. If counting the same type of cell, flush after every 4 or 5 samples and before counting a new cell type.

   The flushing stopcock (in open or vertical position) in combination with the vacuum control stopcock (in open or vertical position) creates a vacuum which flushes out the aperture tube with fresh Isoton. To stop flushing action, both stopcocks must be in closed (horizontal) position. The flushing stopcock must be in closed (horizontal) position while performing the count.

   The manner of opening and closing the stopcocks must be precise; otherwise air will be drawn into the aperture tube. To flush, open flushing stopcock first, then vacuum control stopcock, and flush for 5–10 sec. To stop flushing action, close vacuum control stopcock first, then flushing stopcock. At end of the day, before shutdown, flush aperture tube with Isoterge, a detergent, in a similar manner, leaving the Isoterge in overnight. Then flush with Isoton just prior to resuming counting.

6. **Vacuum Pump.**—The vacuum pump controls the mercury level in the manometer. The vacuum limit of the pump is adjusted by a piece of rubber tubing attached to the pump and pinched off at a predetermined length. This length should not be changed once it has been set.

7. **Vacuum Waste Flask.**—The flask is located on the side of the instrument and connected to the vacuum pump and the top of the control piece by rubber tubing. The flask collects the waste during the flushing of the aperture tube. Make sure fluid in waste flask is below the outflow tube. If level gets too high, it will be drawn into the vacuum pump.

F. Hematocrit Computer

The computer computes the packed red cell volume directly in percentage.

G. Mean Corpuscular Volume Computer

The computer computes the average volume of red cells directly in cubic microns (μ^3).

H. Counting Corrections

1. **Correction for Background.**—Before samples are counted a background count is performed on the Isoton only. This ensures that the Isoton is relatively free of particles. Background counts between 20 and 200/0.5 ml can be disregarded. If the background is sizeable, this must be subtracted from the count of the sample.

2. **Correction for Coincidence Loss.**—Coincidence occurs when two or more cells enter the aperture at the same time and are registered as a single count. To deal with coincidence losses apply coincidence correction factor. Amount of coincidence can be calculated, but reference to the coincidence correction chart allows correction to be made easily. To correct for coincidence read the numbers off the first three glow tubes, refer to the chart and report the corrected count. Correction for coincidence is made for all counts over 10,000. Red cell counts are always corrected for coincidence; white cell counts are corrected if over 10,000. The count loss for coincidence is a function of the aperture's diameter and cell concentration.

VI. PROCEDURE OF COULTER COUNTING

A. Background Count

After a warm-up period, perform a background count.

B. Standard Count

The standards are diluted in the same manner as the samples.

1. **Pfizer Standards.**—These are synthetic standards which have a relatively long expiration date. The values of the standards are printed on the box.

    a. **Celltrol.**—Red blood cell standard; has normal and low abnormal values.

    b. **Leukotrol.**—White blood cell standard; has normal and high abnormal values.

    c. **Globintrol.**—Hemoglobin standard; has normal and low abnormal values.

2. **Coulter 4C.**—This standard has a short expiration date. Coulter 4C is standardized blood for red cells, white cells, hemoglobin and hematocrit. The 4C standards have normal and abnormal values and are accompanied by an assay sheet.

C. Samples of Unknowns

The unknown samples are diluted as described previously (section III. A and B): white cell dilution 1:500, red cell dilution 1:50,000. Each sample should be counted twice and the results averaged. For the white cell count, the duplicate counts on each sample should be within 100 counts of each other. For the red cell count, the duplicate counts on each sample should be within 10,000 counts of each other.

Count the red cells within 10 min after making the dilution, otherwise the cells swell and hemolyze. Count white cells within 30 min after addition of saponin; beyond 30 min the white cells begin to lyse with saponin. Without added saponin white cells in Isoton can stand 4 hr without deterioration.

In counting several samples, count all the red cell samples first, flush aperture tube out with fresh Isoton, then count all the white cell samples. The reason is that the red cell samples contain no saponin and thus will not be hemolyzed.

NOTE: Other systems for automatic cell counting exist, such as Hemalog (Technicon Corp.), Autocytometer (Fisher), Royco Model 920-A, etc. Information regarding these systems can be obtained from the manufacturers.

PROGRAMMED QUESTIONS

Cover answers with a piece of paper. Answers appear at end of questions.

(1) What is the principle upon which the Coulter Counter is based?
   (a) Cells suspended in an electrolyte are poor conductors of electric current
   (b) Voltage drops must be of threshold size to register as a count
   (c) Cells, which are poor conductors of electricity, as they pass through the aperture momentarily decrease electric current, producing a voltage drop
   (d) The mercury manometer uses a vacuum to create a syphon

(2) Which type of anticoagulated venipuncture blood may not be used in the Coulter automatic cell counting procedure?
   (a) Oxalated
   (b) EDTA
   (c) Saponin
   (d) Heparinized

(3) Which component of the Coulter Counter allows one to check on size and size distribution of the cells?
   (a) Aperture control
   (b) Debris monitor
   (c) Discriminator dial
   (d) Oscilloscope monitor

(4) While counting in the Model F Counter Counter, in what position must the flushing stopcock always be?
   (a) Horizontal
   (b) Vertical
   (c) Diagonal
   (d) It does not matter

(5) What range of background counts can be disregarded?
(a) 5–50/mm^3
(b) 20–200/mm^3
(c) 500–1000/mm^3
(d) 300–750/mm^3

(6) What is coincidence count loss?
(a) When 2 or more cells enter the aperture at the same time and are registered as a single count
(b) The first 3 glow tubes refer to the coincidence count loss
(c) Coincidence count loss must be subtracted from background count
(d) When voltage drops are < threshold values

(7) What volume of blood is used in making the dilution of the blood cells for counting in the Model F Coulter Counter?
(a) 10 ml
(b) 0.05 ml
(c) 0.02 ml
(d) 1.0 ml

(8) Within how many minutes must the white cells be counted after the saponin has been added and before the white cells begin to lyse?
(a) 5 min
(b) 10 min
(c) 2 min
(d) 30 min

(9) What is the final dilution of the red blood cells for counting in the Model F Coulter Counter?
(a) 100 times
(b) 50,000 times
(c) 5000 times
(d) 500 times

(10) When the vacuum control stopcock is in the vertical position on the Model F Coulter Counter, _____.
(a) Saline solution flushes the aperture tube
(b) The counting starts as the mercury in the manometer reaches the start electrode
(c) The glow tubes zero as the mercury in the manometer goes below the start electrode
(d) The counting stops as the mercury in the manometer reaches the stop electrode

Answers

(1) c   (6) a
(2) a   (7) c
(3) d   (8) d
(4) a   (9) b
(5) b   (10) c

11

Stained Red Cell Examination

I. SIGNIFICANCE OF STAINED RED CELL EXAMINATION

A. A Distinct Examination from the Differential Count

The stained red cell examination, even though performed on the blood smear of peripheral blood, is a separate and distinct examination from the differential white cell count, but can be done simultaneously as the differential is being counted.

B. Examines the Appearance of Red Cells

The stained red cell examination is to detect the presence of nucleated and abnormal red cells.

II. EXAMINATION AND REPORTING OF NUCLEATED RED CELLS

A. Types of Red Cells

Nucleated red cells are usually confined to the bone marrow, but in anemia and leukemia and after blood dyscrasias (any abnormal or pathologic condition of blood), these cells may appear in the peripheral blood (see Fig. 11.1).

   1. Nucleated Red Cells.—

   Rubriblast.—Mother cell of erythrocytic series

   Characteristics

   a. *Nucleus.*—Large, spherical, centrally located, chromatin network open and fine, 2–5 nucleoli are visible.

   b. *Cytoplasm.*—Contains large quantity of RNA, stains dark blue and is almost homogeneous.

Prorubricyte.—

Characteristics

a.   *Nucleus.*—Centrally located, chromatin network becomes denser and clumps, nucleoli less distinct than previous stage, nucleus is becoming smaller.

b.   *Cytoplasm.*—Contains a large amount of RNA and a small amount of hemoglobin, stains purple-blue to blue (polychromatophilia).

Rubricyte.—

Characteristics

a.   *Nucleus.*—Centrally located, chromatin network continues to clump and becomes denser, nucleoli no longer visible, nucleus becomes smaller, occupies 1/3 cell volume.

b.   *Cytoplasm.*—Due to increased amount of hemoglobin and decreased amount of RNA, stains a grey-blue color (polychromatophilia).

Metarubricyte.—

Characteristics

a.   *Nucleus.*—Centrally located, chromatin network clumped and very dense, nucleus appears as a very small darkly stained sphere (a pyknotic nucleus). The cell loses this nucleus by extrusion.

b.   *Cytoplasm.*—Quite full of hemoglobin with great decrease in amount of RNA, stains pink-tan.

2.   **Nonnucleated Red Cells.—**

a.   **Reticulocyte.**—Cytoplasm nearly full of hemoglobin, but still contains very small amounts of RNA in form of a network or reticulum; stains red-orange. The reticulum of RNA can be observed by supravital staining. The reticulum is lost in 1–2 days.

b.   **Erythrocyte.**—Smooth biconcave structure, cytoplasm full of hemoglobin, contains no RNA, stains red-orange. The erythrocyte is thin in the center where the nucleus was extruded; as there is less hemoglobin here, it stains lighter. The periphery of the cell is thicker. There is more hemoglobin here, so it stains darker.

In summary, as the maturation of the erythrocyte proceeds, the nucleus becomes smaller, denser, and more darkly stained, and ultimately disappears. The cytoplasm, as it accumulates hemoglobin and loses RNA, progressively changes its color on staining from deep blue to grey-blue to reddish. The time for maturation is about 3–5 days, with survival time of the erythrocytes in the peripheral blood between 90 and 120 days, although arguments persist in the literature as to actual life-span of the RBC. The cell also decreases in size as it proceeds toward maturity.

B.   Performing the Nucleated Red Cell Count

Count the number of nucleated red cells seen while performing the differential white cell count, and report as number of nucleated RBC/100 WBC.

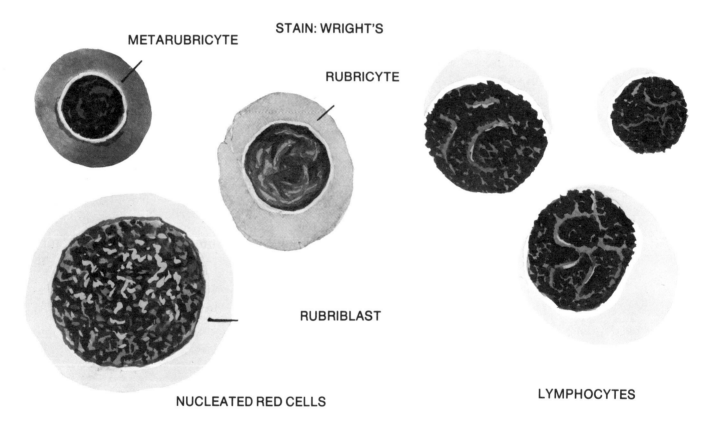

FIG. 11.1. COMPARISON OF NUCLEATED RED CELLS AND LYMPHOCYTES (SEE COLOR ATLAS)

C.   Methods of Identification of Nucleated Red Cells

One must examine cells carefully as some immature forms of nucleated red cells look like small lymphocytes. This can cause some confusion for the inexperienced technician. You can distinguish nucleated red cells from small lymphocytes since the nucleated red cell has a centrally located nucleus, while the lymphocyte nucleus is sometimes eccentrically located. Also, the lymphocyte nucleus occupies almost all of the cell while the RBC nucleus does not. If in doubt, one should seek opinions from fellow technicians and/or the supervisor or hematologist.

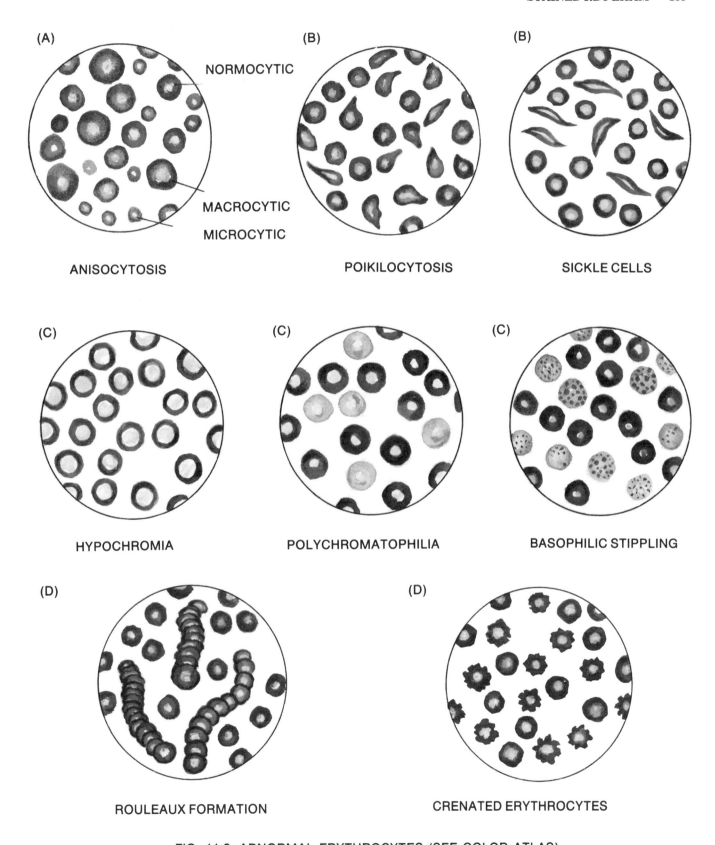

(A)

NORMOCYTIC

MACROCYTIC

MICROCYTIC

ANISOCYTOSIS

(B)

POIKILOCYTOSIS

(B)

SICKLE CELLS

(C)

HYPOCHROMIA

(C)

POLYCHROMATOPHILIA

(C)

BASOPHILIC STIPPLING

(D)

ROULEAUX FORMATION

(D)

CRENATED ERYTHROCYTES

FIG. 11.2. ABNORMAL ERYTHROCYTES (SEE COLOR ATLAS)
(A) Differences in size.
(B) Differences in shape.
(C) Differences in content.
(D) Miscellaneous differences.

III. EXAMINATION AND REPORTING OF ABNORMAL ERYTHROCYTES

A. Types of Abnormal Erythrocytes

There are four groups of abnormal erythrocytes.

1. **Anisocytosis.**—Difference in size—normocytes, microcytes, macrocytes, megalocytes

2. **Poikilocytosis.**—Difference in shape—club, pear, spherical, oval, sickle, target cells

3. **Difference in Cell Content.**—

   a. Hemoglobin content.—Normochromic, hypochromic, hyperchromic
   b. Polychromatophilia.—Cytoplasm of the red cell stains various shades of blue tinged with pink due to presence of RNA and hemoglobin in the cytoplasm.
   c. Basophilic stippling or punctation
   d. Malarial parasites

4. **Miscellaneous Differences.**—

   a. Rouleaux formation
   b. Crenated cells
   c. Partially hemolyzed cells
   d. Poorly stained red cells

B. Performing the Abnormal Red Cell Count (If RBC Abnormalities Are To Be Done Separately)

Using the thin area of the smear where the red cells are uniformly distributed and not overlapping, examine 15 microscopic fields under the oil immersion lens for the abnormal red cells. The three most common abnormalities reported are anisocytosis, poikilocytosis and variation in hemoglobin content (hyperchromia, hypochromia). The abnormalities are reported either as present or absent; or slight, moderate or marked. The latter semiquantitative method is hard for beginners, but one learns to quantitate with experience and with guidance from other laboratory personnel.

C. Method for Identification of Abnormal Erythrocyte from Normal Erythrocyte

Distorted normal erythrocytes can be mistaken for abnormal ones, particularly along edges of the smear. Seek guidance from more experienced laboratorians.

In performing a stained red cell examination, examine the blood smear first for nucleated red cells as you count the differential white cell count. Then examine for abnormal erythrocytes.

PROGRAMMED QUESTIONS

Cover answers with a piece of paper.   Answers appear at end of questions.

(1) Characteristics of the reticulocyte are
_____.
  (a) Has coarse nuclear chromatin net-
      work
  (b) Has several nucleoli
  (c) Nucleus is centrally located in the cell
  (d) None of the above

(2) At what point while performing a CBC is
a nucleated red cell count performed?
  (a) While doing the Fonio indirect plate-
      let count
  (b) While performing the differential
      white cell count
  (c) While examining 15 random micro-
      scopic fields
  (d) While counting reticulocytes

(3) From the list below, which cell exhibits a
grey-blue stained cytoplasm?
  (a) Rubricyte
  (b) Rubriblast
  (c) Lymphocyte
  (d) Erythrocyte

(4) What term describes variation in shape
of erythrocytes?
  (a) Anisocytosis
  (b) Hypochromia
  (c) Poikilocytosis
  (d) Crenation

(5) What is a simple method of identification used to distinguish nucleated red
cells from lymphocytes?
  (a) Lymphocyte nucleus centrally locat-
      ed; nucleated red cell nucleus eccen-
      trically located
  (b) Ratio of nucleus to cytoplasm
  (c) All nucleated red cells have pyknotic
      nuclei
  (d) Nucleated red cells are biconcave-
      shaped cells, while lymphocytes are
      all spherical-shaped cells

(6) What power of the microscope and how
many microscopic fields are examined
when performing a stained red cell examination for abnormal red cells?
  (a) High dry; 15 microscopic fields
  (b) Low; 3 microscopic fields
  (c) Scanning; 10 microscopic fields
  (d) Oil immersion; 15 microscopic fields

(7) What term describes staining of an
erythrocyte that contains both hemoglobin and RNA?
  (a) Polychromatophilia
  (b) Ovalocytosis
  (c) Hyperchromic
  (d) Anisocytosis

(8) What is rouleaux formation?
  (a) Arrangement of abnormal-sized
      erythrocytes
  (b) Arrangement of spherocytes in a
      design pattern
  (c) Arrangement of erythrocytes re-
      sembling a roll of coins
  (d) Arrangement of leukocytes resem-
      bling a roll of coins

(9) Which is the last nucleated red cell in the maturation series to possess a nucleus?
 (a) Reticulocyte
 (b) Metarubricyte
 (c) Rubriblast
 (d) Prorubricyte

(10) If an erythrocyte is macrocytic or microcytic in size relative to a normal-sized erythrocyte, a condition known as _____ exists.
 (a) Basophilic punctation
 (b) Poikilocytosis
 (c) Polychromatophilia
 (d) Anisocytosis

Answers

(1) d	(6) d
(2) b	(7) a
(3) a	(8) c
(4) c	(9) b
(5) b	(10) d

12

Complete Routine Urinalysis—Part I

NOTE: Before beginning the following exercise the student should carefully review the gross and microscopic anatomy and physiology of the kidney from a standard text.

Urine is the most significant way of elimination of <u>nonvolatile</u> substances from the body. These include nitrogenous substances of protein and nucleic acid metabolism, such as urea, uric acid, creatinine; ingested substances, such as excess glucose and water; and substances of cellular metabolism produced in excess, such as water and electrolytes. Carbon dioxide, the main <u>volatile</u> substance, is eliminated by way of the lungs.

The composition of urine reflects the kidneys' function in maintaining homeostasis of the organism. Urine composition will vary widely among individuals of different ages, diet and physical activity. A routine urinalysis usually consists of the following examinations.

A. Physical Tests (Exercise 12)

1. Color
2. Turbidity or physical condition
3. Odor
4. pH or reaction
5. Specific gravity

B. Chemical Tests (Exercise 13)

1. Proteinuria (albumin)
2. Glycosuria (glucose)
3. Ketonuria (diacetic acid or acetone)
4. Bilirubinuria (bile)

C. Microscopic Examination (Exercise 14)

1. Epithelial cells
2. Blood cells (red and white)
3. Casts
4. Bacteria
5. Miscellaneous substances (cylindroids, mucus threads, protozoa, yeast)
6. Crystals and amorphous deposits

Some variation exists depending upon the laboratory.

The following indicates a partial list of some special urinalysis tests.

SPECIAL URINALYSIS TESTS

A. Physical Tests

   1.   **Volume.**—Determined for 12 and 24 hr collections

   2.   **Osmolality**

B. Chemical Tests

   1.   **Protein.—**

   a.   Bence-Jones protein
   b.   Specific amino acids or their metabolic products, such as phenylpyruvic acid, homogentisic acid, urea, uric acid, ammonia, creatinine, creatine

   2.   **Carbohydrates.—**

   a.   Specific sugars besides glucose
   b.   Mucopolysaccharides

   3.   **Hemoglobin.—**Its products of degradation, its precursor molecules

   a.   Hematuria (occult blood) or hemoglobinuria (free hemoglobin)
   b.   Urobilinogen
   c.   Porphobilinogen and other tests for precursor molecules of hemoglobin
   d.   Myoglobin

   4.   **Calcium**

C. Microscopic Examination

   1.   Crystals of amino acids
   2.   Lipids—cholesterol
   3.   Drugs

I.   COLLECTING URINE SAMPLES

Urine samples are collected in clean vessels; there should be no residue from previous use. It is preferable to use clean disposable plastic vessels, which indeed is current practice.

A. Random Sample

This sample is of no particular value in giving accurate information of the urinary character of the person because there are transitory increases of substances in the urine due to eating.

B. Twelve Hour Sample

The urine is collected either from 8 a.m. to 8 p.m. (day sample) or 8 p.m. to 8 a.m. (night sample). The day-night samples check for pathological conditions.

C. Twenty-four Hour Sample

The 24 hr sample is important when quantitative studies are necessary, as for sugar and albumin excretion. Instructions to the patient must be exact, otherwise a true 24 hr sample will not be obtained and high values will result. Instruct patient to empty bladder at 8 a.m., discard urine, then collect all urine from that time up to and including urine voided at 8 a.m. the next day. Mix together all urine voided. Keep urine under refrigeration in a stoppered bottle. A sample of the 24 hr collection is taken for analysis. Some laboratories add a preservative to the urine (see below).

D. First Morning Sample or A.M. Sample

Discard voided urine before retiring, then collect the first urine sample on getting out of bed in the morning. This is the preferred sample for routine urinalysis. This sample represents a long period of uniform excretion of urine of sufficient volume and concentration. In this sample there is little tendency to have a transitory increase in various substances due to eating as would be characteristic of a random sample.

E. Catheterized Sample

This sample is used when utmost accuracy or sterility (as for culturing) is required.

II. PRESERVATION OF URINE SAMPLES

The samples should be examined, if possible, within 30 min after collection. If samples cannot be examined immediately, a preservative or refrigeration should be utilized. There are several ways to preserve the urine.

A. Refrigeration

Refrigerate sample at 0°–4°C. (This tends to cause precipitation of certain crystals which might obscure microscopic examination.)

B. Addition of Bacterial Inhibitors

1. **Formalin or Thymol.**—These will inhibit bacterial growth, but they do not interfere with tests of urinary constituents. A few drops of 10% formalin or a thymol crystal is usually sufficient.

2. **Toluene.**—Overlay urine with a thin layer of toluene. This excludes air (oxygen) from urine sample and inhibits aerobic bacterial growth. Preservation of urine samples suppresses growth of bacteria, prevents breakdown of solutes in the urine and breakdown of urinary sediments. Since the preservatives suppress bacterial growth, the conversion of urea to ammonia and degradation of glucose is decreased. Furthermore, since bacterial growth is inhibited, the possibility of bacterial proteins' interfering with the protein test is diminished. Since there is little conversion of urea to ammonia, the preservative maintains the acid pH of the urine. The preservative may increase the specific gravity of the urine but the preservative should not interfere with the other tests performed on the urine.

III. EXAMINATION OF URINE SAMPLES

There are three general approaches used in performing routine urinalysis. By these routine procedures normal and abnormal renal function can be estimated.
A. Physicochemical or physical tests
B. Chemical screening tests
C. Microscopic examination of urinary sediments

A. Physicochemical or Physical Tests

1. **Volume.**—1000–2000 ml/24 hr are excreted, with the average value 1500 ml/24 hr. Volume varies with diet, fluid intake, temperature and physical activity. The day volume is 2–4 times that of the night volume.

   a. **Diuresis.**—Any increase in urine volume output above normal

   b. **Polyuria.**—A large increase in urine volume output above normal

   c. **Oliguria.**—A decrease in urine volume output below normal

   d. **Anuria.**—A complete lack of urine volume output

2. **Color of Urine.**—Normal color of urine is straw, yellow or amber. The color is due to normal metabolic degradation products of hemoglobin, such as urochrome and urobilin, and concentration of these solutes. Under abnormal conditions or medication, the color of urine may vary from red through bright yellow, green, orange, brown or black.

3. **Turbidity or Physical Condition.**—Normal urine is perfectly clear and transparent on first being voided. On standing for a variable period of time, the urine becomes cloudy due to normal precipitation of certain urinary constituents or bacterial proliferation.

   Freshly voided turbid urine arises from pathological conditions or from the presence of various crystals or bacteria in large numbers.

4. **Odor.**—Normal urine has a faint aromatic odor due to volatile organic acids in the urine. The normal odor of urine changes on intake of specific types of drugs or foods into the body. On standing, urine takes on an ammoniacal odor due to bacterial decomposition of urea to ammonia.

$$\text{Urea} \xrightarrow[\text{decomposition}]{\text{bacterial}} NH_3\uparrow$$

5. **pH or Reaction.**—pH of the urine reflects the kidneys' ability to maintain normal H^+ ion concentration in the plasma and extracellular fluids of the body. The normal pH of the urine is 6.0, slightly acidic, with a range of 4.6–8.0.

The slightly acidic pH of the urine is maintained as follows. As a result of cellular metabolic activity, sodium salts of various acids are produced (Na_2SO_4, Na_3PO_4, $NaCl$). Since the body cannot tolerate a great loss of Na^+, the kidney conserves Na^+ and exchanges the Na^+ with H^+. The free H^+ ions would make the urine very acidic; however, the H^+ ions are buffered by NH_3, produced by the cells of the distal convoluted tubules of the kidney nephron, which forms ammonium ions (NH_4^+).

$$NH_3 + H^+ \longrightarrow NH_4^+$$

The NH_4^+ ions are excreted as ammonium salts. The free H^+ ions, which are not buffered, are excreted and make the urine only slightly acidic. The pH is measured by litmus paper, phenolphthalein, nitrazine pH indicator paper, Hydrion pH indicator paper, or a pH meter with glass electrode. The indicator papers are impregnated with a dye indicator. Hydrion paper is the most popular in current usage. The indicator is a salt of a weak acid or base and exhibits one color when the salt is nonionized and another color in the ionized form. The nonionized and ionized forms of the indicator depend on the pH of the solution into which they are placed. Thus by the color of the indicator, the approximate pH can be estimated. The pH meter with glass electrode allows for a more accurate determination of pH but is seldom used routinely.

6. **Specific Gravity.**—Specific gravity of a solution is the ratio of the weight of a specific volume of the solution (urine) to the weight of an equal volume of pure distilled water, both measured at the same specified temperature (4°C).

$$\text{sp. gy. of urine} = \frac{\text{weight of a specific volume of urine at 4°C}}{\text{weight of an equal volume of distilled } H_2O \text{ at 4°C}}$$

Normal specific gravity (isosthenuria) varies from 1.010–1.022, with wide variation above and below the indicated range still considered as normal. When the specific gravity of urine is low (hyposthenuria) the values are less than 1.007. When the specific gravity of urine is high (hypersthenuria) the values are 1.030 or higher.

Specific gravity of urine is a measure of the total amount of solute in a specific volume, or total urine solute concentration. Specific gravity generally varies inversely with volume. Specific gravity is a measure of the kidney's concentrating or diluting powers as reflected in the total amount of solute excreted. The specific gravity increases with increased amounts of solute in the urine, but increase in specific gravity is not the same for every kind of solute in solution as some solutes are ionized and others are not. Urea, chloride, sulfate, and phosphate ions contribute most to the specific gravity of the urine. The amount of urea in the urine reflects the amount of protein in the diet; the quantity of Cl⁻ ions in the urine reflects amount of salt in the diet.

a. Measurement of Specific Gravity (See Fig. 12.1).—

(1) *Urinometer or Hydrometer.*—This measures specific gravity at room temperature. Have urine come to room temperature and mix urine well. Fill urinometer vessel with about 15 ml of urine. Insert urinometer float with a spinning motion so that it will float free. The float must not touch bottom or side walls of vessel. Read the calibrations on the float at the meniscus of the urine as 1.0--. The lower the float sinks, the less dense the urine, and the closer the urine is to pure distilled water and a reading of 1.000. The higher the float rises, the more concentrated the urine.

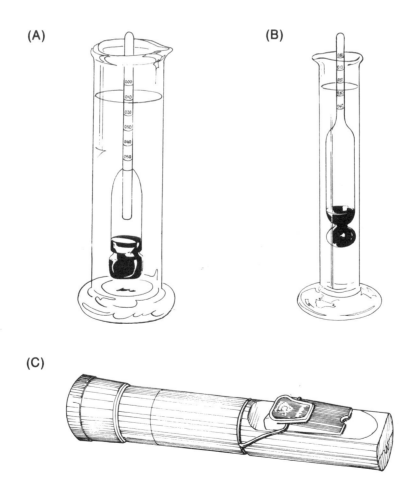

(A)

(B)

(C)

FIG. 12.1. INSTRUMENTS USED TO MEASURE SPECIFIC GRAVITY
(A) Regular urinometer.
(B) Midget urinometer.
(C) Refractometer.

Sources of Error in Urinometer Measurement of Urinary Specific Gravity

- (a) Temperature.—Urinometers are calibrated at 20°C. A change of 3°C between urine temperature and calibration temperature requires a 0.001 correction.
- (b) Protein.—1% protein in the urine increases the specific gravity 0.003 and should be corrected.
- (c) Glucose.—1% glucose in the urine increases the specific gravity 0.004 and should be corrected.
- (d) Some urinary preservatives increase specific gravity.
- (e) X-ray contrast media increase specific gravity.

(2) *Refractometer.*—This uses a small volume of urine (1 drop) (see Fig. 12.1). Place 1 drop of urine on the refractometer's platform, cover and press gently to uniformly distribute the urine on the platform. Hold the refractometer to your eye toward a light source either horizontally or at a downward slant. Adjust eyepiece so as to read scale. The reading is made from within the eyepiece at the meniscus of the urine. The refractive index reading of the scale is converted to urinary specific gravity by comparison with the conversion table. Some refractometers are calibrated directly in specific gravity.

Refractive index is the ratio of the velocity of light in air to velocity of light in a solution. The ratio varies directly to the number of dissolved particles in the solution and correlates closely with specific gravity of a solution.

7. **Osmolality.**—Osmolality is a more accurate measure of solute content than specific gravity. Osmolality is a measure of the number of particles of solute in a given weight of solvent.

Osmolality is measured by freezing point depression or vapor pressure elevation of a solution, using either a freezing point osmometer or vapor pressure osmometer.

PROGRAMMED QUESTIONS

Cover answers with a piece of paper.   Answers appear at end of questions.

(1) Which urine sample is best to collect for routine urinalysis?
   (a) Random sample
   (b) 24 hr sample
   (c) 12 hr sample
   (d) A.M. sample

(2) As a result of cell metabolism, which of the following is a nonvolatile substance that is eliminated from the body by way of the kidney?
   (a) Uric acid
   (b) Glucose
   (c) Carbon dioxide
   (d) Protein

(3) A large increase in urine volume output above normal is termed _____.
   (a) Oliguria
   (b) Polyuria
   (c) Diuresis
   (d) Anuria

(4) What is the normal pH for freshly voided urine?
   (a) pH 3–4
   (b) pH 4–5
   (c) pH 5–6
   (d) pH 2–3

(5) When measuring specific gravity with a urinometer, the lower the float sinks, _____.
   (a) The closer the urine is to distilled water
   (b) The more light is refracted
   (c) The more concentrated the urine is
   (d) The more the freezing point is depressed

(6) Which of the following should be used to preserve urine samples if they cannot be examined within 30 min of collection?
   (a) Addition of ammonia
   (b) Treatment with X-ray
   (c) Overlayer of toluene
   (d) Incubation at 37°C

(7) From the list below, choose the substance that gives the normal color to urine.
   (a) Bacteria
   (b) Hemoglobin
   (c) Organic acids
   (d) Urobilin

(8) Crystals are normally not present in freshly voided urine, but form as the urine _____.
   (a) Becomes alkaline on standing
   (b) Cools to room temperature
   (c) Specific gravity increases
   (d) Is shaken before analysis

(9) Complete the equation:

$$\text{urea} \xrightarrow[\text{decomposition}]{\text{bacterial}} \underline{\hspace{2cm}}$$

   (a) NH_3
   (b) NH_4^+
   (c) CO_2
   (d) Uric acid

(10) What substance buffers most of the free H^+ ion in the kidney?
   (a) NH_4^+
   (b) Urea
   (c) NH_3
   (d) NaCl

Answers

(1) d	(6) c
(2) a	(7) d
(3) b	(8) b
(4) c	(9) a
(5) a	(10) c

13

Complete Routine Urinalysis—Part II

B. Chemical Screening Tests

The chemical screening tests when properly executed will indicate the presence of renal disease and urinary tract infections, as well as diabetes mellitus, jaundice, phenylketonuria, etc.

The chemical screening tests are usually performed after one has completed the physical tests and during the time the urine is centrifuging for the microscopic examination.

These chemical tests screen the urine samples for presence or absence of various substances and semiquantitate the approximate amount of the substances. Most of the chemical screening tests used are reagents in tablet form or test strips of plastic impregnated with the reagent. The Ames Company strips are widely used. But historical, accurate older methods are still in common usage.

1. **Reagent Strip Method.—**

    a. **Use of the Test Strips.—**

    (1) Dip test area of strip into well mixed urine. Test area of the strip must be completely moistened. Remove immediately; do not dip excessively, otherwise reagent on strip will leach out.

    (2) Touch strip to edge of vessel containing the urine to drain excess urine.

    (3) Compare color of test area of strip to the color chart on the bottle. Observe time for reading each strip. Hold test area of strip close to color chart; read under good lighting conditions from color chart to test area of strip.

    b. **Precautions To Take with Test Strips.—**

    (1) Protect strips from moisture and heat; store strips in cool, dry place, but not in the refrigerator.

    (2) Brownish discoloration indicates significant loss of reactivity.

    (3) Remove only enough strips for immediate use, tightly recap bottle immediately.

    (4) Avoid contamination of test area of strip; place strips on a clean sheet of paper, not directly on the table top.

    (5) Do not use strips in presence of acid or alkali fumes, which will inactivate the test area of the strip.

    (6) Note expiration date on strip container.

2. **Proteinuria.**—Proteinuria is an increased amount of protein in urine. The proteinuria is usually due to albumin in the urine, so the condition is also known as albuminuria.

    a. **Albustix.**—The colorimetric reagent strip screening test for albumin in the urine is albustix.

        (1) *Theory.*—This is a colorimetric test based upon proteins' ability to change the color of an acid-base indicator without a change in pH. At a particular pH (pH 3) the indicator dye, tetrabromphenol blue, is yellow in the absence of protein, whereas in the presence of protein, the indicator will be green through blue depending on amount of protein present.

        (2) *Method.*—Dip test area of strip into urine, drain excess urine, immediately compare color developed on the test area of the strip to color chart on the bottle.

        (3) *Interpretation.*—Negative test: no color change in test area of strip. Positive test: if protein is present, test area of strip changes from yellow to yellow-green, green or blue-green depending on quantity of protein present. Report results as negative, trace, 1+ to 4+. The 1+ to 4+ gives the approximate concentration of protein in mg/100 ml urine.

        (4) *Sensitivity.*—Any urinary screening test should not be too sensitive, as it is required to differentiate normal amounts of excreted substance from abnormal amounts. Eight to 10 mg protein/100 ml urine is normally present in the urine; this amount is not detected by albustix. The sensitivity of the albustix detects 20–30 mg protein/100 ml urine. The test is more sensitive to albumin than to globulin.

        (5) *Specificity.*—The reagent of the albustix is not affected by other urinary constituents or drugs. Decomposed or highly buffered alkaline urine which is free of protein may give a false positive reaction due to pH change with the acid-base indicator dye. A false positive reaction means test is positive, although the substance in question is not present. Something else in the urine is causing the test to be positive. All positive screening tests should be verified by another method.

    b. **Sulfosalicylic Acid Protein Test.**—

        (1) *Theory.*—This screening test relies on the precipitation of protein without heating. The sulfosalicylic acid denatures the protein so that it becomes less soluble and is precipitated in the urine with turbidity or cloudiness approximately proportional to the concentration of the protein.

        (2) *Method.*—

            (a) If urine is turbid, clear the urine by centrifugation.
            (b) Into a test tube place 3–5 ml of clear urine.
            (c) Add to the urine a few drops of a 20% solution of sulfosalicylic acid. (Some laboratories prefer a 10% or 12% solution.)

(3) *Interpretation.*—Negative test: if no protein is present, no turbidity is observed. Positive test: if protein is present, a cloudy precipitate will appear. Report results as negative, faint trace, trace, or 1+ to 4+. A 4+ appears like solid egg white.

(4) *Sensitivity.*—This test is extremely sensitive; it can pick up protein as small as 0.25 mg/100 ml urine.

(5) *Specificity.*—This test may give false positive tests with many drugs and many normal urinary constituents. If the urine is alkaline, the test may give a false negative result. This would mean the protein is present, but the alkaline pH prevents the precipitate from forming. However, it is highly reliable and is frequently used to back up a positive "dip-stick" result.

3.   **Glycosuria or Glucosuria.**—The routine screening of the urine sample for glucose is primarily to detect diabetes mellitus. However, there are other causative factors that may lead to reducing sugars' being present in the urine. Several methods for determining glucose in the urine are in current use.

a.   **Qualitative Benedict's Test.—**

(1) *Theory.*—The classical method for measuring glucose and other reducing sugars in the urine is based upon the chemical reaction that molecules with free ketone $(C=O)$ or aldehyde groups $(H-C=O)$ when heated with Benedict's solution can reduce an alkaline, blue cupric (Cu^{++}) sulfate solution $(CuSO_4)$ to a red cuprous (Cu^{+}) oxide (Cu_2O) precipitate.

$$\text{cupric sulfate} + \text{reducing sugar} \longrightarrow \text{cuprous oxide} + \text{oxidized sugar}$$

$$\begin{array}{ccc} (Cu^{++}) & & (Cu^{+}) \\ \text{(alkaline blue solution)} & & \text{(red precipitate)} \end{array}$$

Reducing sugars have free ketone or aldehyde groups.

(2) *Method.—*

(a)   Place 5 ml of Benedict's qualitative reagent into a test tube.
(b)   Add 0.5 ml or 8 drops of urine; mix.
(c)   Place test tube in boiling water bath for 3–5 min.
(d)   Remove, swirl contents, read the results.

(3) *Interpretation.*—Depending on amount of sugar in the urine, a graded series of colors from blue, which is negative, to brick red, which indicates approximately 3–4% sugar, is obtained (see Table 13.1).

(4) *Sensitivity.*—Test is sensitive between 50–80 mg glucose/100 ml urine. Less than this amount in the urine will not be picked up by the test. Normal individuals are negative as a total of only 130 mg glucose is usually excreted in a 24 hr period.

TABLE 13.1

INTERPRETATION OF BENEDICT'S TEST

Color	Report As	Approximate Amount of Glucose
Clear blue	negative	0–0.25%
Clear green	faint trace	0–0.25%
Green opacity, no precipitate	trace	0.25–0.50%
Green with yellow precipitate	1+	0.50%
Yellow with green-yellow precipitate	2+	0.75–2.0%
Orange with yellow precipitate	3+	2.0–3.0%
Orange or red with brick-red precipitate	4+	3.0% and over

(5) *Specificity.*—The qualitative Benedict's test is not a very specific test for glucosuria, since other reducing sugars also give positive tests, such as fructose, galactose, lactose, maltose, pentose. Other urinary constituents, drugs and contaminants in the urine may give false positive results.

b. Clinitest Tablet.—

(1) *Theory.*—This is a single tablet copper reduction test, which is a modification of Benedict's qualitative test, i.e., it is a Benedict's test in pill form which incorporates NaOH to accomplish boiling.

(2) *Method.—*

(a) Place 5 drops of urine into a test tube

(b) Add 10 drops of distilled water

(c) Add 1 Clinitest tablet

Reaction will boil; do not shake during this time.

(d) After boiling has stopped, shake gently; compare color obtained to the color chart.

(3) *Interpretation.*—Same as for Benedict's qualitative test; report results as negative, faint trace, trace, 1+ to 4+.

(4) *Sensitivity.*—Clinitest is less sensitive to reducing substances in the urine than Benedict's qualitative test.

(5) *Specificity.*—Clinitest is not affected by normal urinary constituents. Drugs in high amounts will give false positive reactions.

NOTE: Tablets must be fresh and stored in tightly capped bottles. If pills have turned greyish with black dots they are spoiled. Some laboratories prefer to use individually foil-wrapped tablets to prevent this.

c. Glucose Oxidase Test—Clinistix

(1) *Theory.*—This is an enzymatic method specific only for glucose. Other reducing sugars which are not substrates for the enzyme do not react. The reaction is an enzymatic oxidation: the glucose in the urine is oxidized to gluconic acid by glucose oxidase.

$$\text{glucose} + O_2 \xrightarrow[\text{oxidase}]{\text{glucose}} \text{gluconic acid} + H_2O_2$$

Hydrogen removed in the oxidation of the glucose combines with oxygen to form hydrogen peroxide. The hydrogen peroxide in the presence of another enzyme, peroxidase, oxidizes the dye orthotoluidine (alternate spelling—orthotolidine), which is red, to oxidized orthotoluidine, which is purple-blue, plus water.

$$H_2O_2 + \underset{\text{(red)}}{\text{reduced orthotoluidine}} \xrightarrow{\text{peroxidase}} \underset{\text{(purple-blue)}}{\text{oxidized orthotoluidine}} + H_2O$$

The test is simplified by test area of clinistix's being impregnated with glucose oxidase, peroxidase, and orthotoluidine.

(2) *Method.*—

(a) Dip test area of clinistix into well-mixed urine; remove immediately.
(b) Drain excess urine.
(c) Wait 10 sec for color development; compare test area of strip to color chart. Color development within 10 sec is considered a positive test; however, a 1 min wait should be allowed for color development.

(3) *Interpretation.*—Negative test: test area remains red. Positive test: test area becomes purple. Light purple, small amount of glucose; dark purple, large amount of glucose. The quantitation is not accurate.

(4) *Sensitivity.*—The enzymatic test is most sensitive, as it can detect as little as 0.01%–0.1% glucose.

(5) *Specificity.*—The glucose oxidase test is specific for glucose only; since it is an enzymatic test, no other reducing sugar affects the test. Normal urinary constituents and drugs have no effect on the test. The test works well over a wide pH range between 5 and 9. Large quantities of ascorbic acid will suppress color development. If a patient is taking ascorbic acid or ascorbic acid-containing drugs, wait 2 or more minutes before reading the test as negative.

Diastix and ketodiastix are similar to clinistix in their method of action, but a different dye is used.

The use of copper reduction tests in combination with the enzymatic test can help to identify if the reducing sugar is glucose.

(a)   The copper reduction test is used to establish the presence of a reducing substance.

(b)   The enzymatic test is used to identify glucose.

If tests (a) and (b) are positive, the reducing sugar is specifically glucose. If test (a) is positive and test (b) is negative, the reducing substance is not glucose. To further identify other reducing sugars, methods for specific reducing substances must be employed (see any standard text).

4.   **Ketonuria.**—A defect in carbohydrate metabolism leads to improper fat metabolism thus causing fat to be incompletely metabolized to ketone bodies. Under normal carbohydrate metabolism fats are completely oxidized to carbon dioxide and water. The ketone bodies appear in the blood (ketonemia) and are then excreted in the urine (ketonuria). The three ketone bodies are acetoacetic acid (diacetic acid) 20%, acetone 2%, β-hydroxybutyric acid (β-OH) 78%. Acetone is volatile and is mainly lost by way of the lungs; the other two ketones are lost by way of the urine.

Since ketonuria is nonspecific, as all three are excreted in the urine, any test procedure which determines one of these three components would be satisfactory for the diagnosis of ketonuria. The tests are mainly for acetoacetic acid and less so for acetone or β-hydroxybutyric acid.

a.   **Rothera–Lange Nitroferricyanide or Nitroprusside Test.**—This is the classical test to demonstrate the presence of ketone bodies. The test is 20 times more sensitive to acetoacetic acid than to acetone.

(1)   *Theory.*—The nitroferricyanide reacts with the acetoacetic acid in the presence of alkali to produce a purple-colored complex.

(2)   *Method.*—

(a)   Rothera's Test

(a-1) Place 5 ml of fresh urine into a test tube.

(a-2) Add 5–8 drops (0.5 ml) of glacial acetic acid.

(a-3) Add 2–4 drops of Rothera's reagent (a supersaturated solution of sodium nitroferricyanide or nitroprusside).

(a-4) Layer over the urine 5 ml of concentrated NH_4OH. Allow NH_4OH to flow gently down side of inclined test tube.

(a-5) If ketones are present, a pink-purple ring develops at interface between urine and NH_4OH within 1.5 min.

(b)   Alternative Rothera's Test

(b-1) Place 5 ml of fresh urine in a test tube.

(b-2) Add 3–5 drops of Rothera's reagent.

(b-3) Add 1 ml of 10% monoethanolamine; mix well.

(b-4) If ketones are present, purple color will develop within 1.5 min.

Interpretation.—Negative test: no color or brown color development. Positive test: pink-purple, color development rated as faint trace, trace, 2+ to 4+ (small, moderate, large). A 4+ is a deep purple-violet color.

(4) *Sensitivity.*—Test is very sensitive as it picks up very small amounts of ketone in the urine.

(5) *Specificity.*—Test is non-specific as acetoacetic acid, acetone and β-hydroxybutyric acid will give positive tests.

b. **Ketostix.**—This is a modification of the Rothera-Lange Procedure, as the Rothera's reagent is impregnated into the test area of the strip.

   (1) *Theory.*—The ketones form a purple-colored complex with Rothera's reagent.

   (2) *Method.*—

   (a) Dip test area of strip into fresh urine; drain excess urine.
   (b) After 15 sec compare test area of strip to color chart.

   (3) *Interpretation.*—Negative test: color of test area remains buff color. Positive test: intensity of purple color proportional to quantity of ketone bodies present; lavender, small amount; purple, large amount.

   (4) *Sensitivity.*—Reacts with acetoacetic acid at 5–10 mg/100 ml urine. Test is less sensitive to acetone.

   (5) *Specificity.*—Test is not specific as acetoacetic acid and acetone both give positive tests. β-Hydroxybutyric acid will not react with this test. Certain drugs may give false positives, as may excretion of large concentrations of phenylketones.

c. **Acetest Tablet.—**

   (1) *Theory.*—The test is the same as the Rothera-Lange procedure, but test is packaged as a tablet.

   (2) *Method.*—

   (a) Place an acetest tablet on a piece of supplied filter paper pad.
   (b) Place 1 drop of fresh urine on the tablet.
   (c) After 30 sec compare test to color chart.

   (3) *Interpretation.*—Same as ketostix.

   (4) *Sensitivity.*—Detects 5 mg acetoacetic acid/100 ml urine or less.

   (5) *Specificity.*—Same as ketostix.

d. **Stability of Ketones.**—Freshly voided urine contains more ketone bodies than urine that has been standing around. On standing, bacteria convert acetoacetic acid to acetone, which is a volatile substance and evaporates from the urine at room temperature. If urine cannot be immediately tested, it should be placed in a tightly closed container and refrigerated until use.

5. **Bilirubinuria—Ictotest.**—These tests determine if bilirubin is in the urine. Bilirubin is a degradation product of hemoglobin. Bilirubin is present in the urine in several liver disorders or in the common bile duct obstruction, obstructive jaundice. A positive bili-

rubin test appears in the urine even before any sign of jaundice is apparent. Bilirubinuria is an important diagnostic sign of liver disease.

a. Ictotest (Diazo Test).—

(1) *Theory.*—The Ictotest tablet or Ictostix contains a diazo dye which couples with bilirubin on addition of water to form a blue to purple-colored complex.

(2) *Method for Ictotest Tablet.*—

(a) Place 5 drops of urine on the asbestos-cellulose mat. If bilirubin is present, it will be absorbed on the mat surface.
(b) Place an Ictotest tablet on moistened area of mat.
(c) Place 2 drops of water on tablet to dissolve some of the tablet and to wash contents of the tablet onto the mat.
(d) Wait 30 sec.

(3) *Interpretation.*—Negative test: mat around tablet shows no blue or purple color within 30 sec. Pink or red color on mat is a negative test. Positive test: mat around tablet turns blue or purple. Speed and intensity of color development is proportional to amount of bilirubin in the urine.

(4) *Sensitivity.*—Test is sensitive to 0.1 mg/100 ml urine. Normal amounts of bilirubin (0.02 mg/100 ml of urine) in the urine give a negative test.

(5) *Specificity.*—The test is specific only for bilirubin; other usual urinary constituents of normal urine will not react with the diazo dye. Many drugs cause color changes in the urine. Diazo test will give a false negative if the bilirubin is oxidized to biliverdin. Urine should be examined within one week of collection as bilirubin is not stable in the urine in the presence of light and is converted to biliverdin.

b. Fouchet Test (Oxidation Test).—

(1) *Theory.*—The colorless bilirubin is oxidized by the ferric ion of ferric chloride to green biliverdin.

$$\text{bilirubin} + Fe^{+++} \longrightarrow \text{biliverdin} + Fe^{++}$$
$$\text{(colorless)} \qquad\qquad\qquad \text{(green)}$$

Barium chloride is added to urine to precipitate urinary phosphates as barium phosphate. Bilirubin is adsorbed to the barium phosphate surface and then is oxidized by the ferric chloride of Fouchet reagent.

(2) *Method.*—

(a) To 10 ml of acidified urine add 5 ml of 10% barium chloride; shake and filter through filter paper.
(b) Spread filter paper out and when partly dry add 1–2 drops of Fouchet's reagent to the residual precipitate. Fouchet's reagent consists of

Trichloroacetic acid	25 g
10% Ferric chloride	10 ml
Distilled water	100 ml

(3) *Interpretation.*—Negative test: no color change. Positive test: various shades of green depending on amount of biliverdin present indicate bilirubin in the urine. Report result as trace, 1+ to 4+.

(4) *Sensitivity.*—Test is sensitive to 0.05–0.1 mg/100 ml urine. Normal amount of bilirubin in urine gives a negative test.

(5) *Specificity.*—Not as specific as the diazo test. Many drugs cause color changes, and high levels of urobilin and urobilinogen cause brown to red color which could mask the green of the biliverdin.

6.   **Urobilinogen in the Urine.**—Urobilinogen is a breakdown product of bilirubin. Normally urine contains a small or trace amount of urobilinogen and its oxidized form, urobilin. Increase in urinary urobilinogen occurs when there is increased destruction of red cells as in hemolytic anemias or in certain liver diseases. Urobilinogen tests in combination with test for bilirubinuria can distinguish various types of liver diseases, hemolytic diseases and bile duct obstruction. For example, a negative test for urobilinogen and a positive test for bilirubin indicate bile duct obstruction. In hemolytic anemias, urobilinogen gives a positive test, while bilirubin gives a negative test.

Relationship Between Urinary Bilirubin and Urobilinogen

	Urine Bilirubin	Urine Urobilinogen
Normal	absent	trace
Hepatitis	increased	increased
Bile duct obstruction	increased	absent
Hemolytic anemia	absent	increased
Impaired liver function	absent	increased

a. **Urobilistix.—**

(1) *Theory.*—Dimethylaminobenzaldehyde in an acidic buffered solution is impregnated onto the urobilistix. Urobilinogen or other similar molecules react with dimethylaminobenzaldehyde to form red-colored molecules.

(2) *Method.*—

(a) Dip test area of urobilistix into freshly voided urine collected between 2 and 4 p.m. when urobilinogen is thought to be highest for the day.

(b) Drain excess urine.

(c) Wait 60 sec; compare color of test area to color chart.

(3) *Interpretation.*—Negative test: test area remains bright yellow. Negative test is not accurate to detect an absence of urobilinogen. Positive test: depending

upon how much urobilinogen is present, color changes from yellow through various shades of red through brown.

(4) *Sensitivity.*—Detects > 4 mg of urobilinogen/24 hr. Normally, excretion of urobilinogen is 0.5–2.5 mg/24 hr, so this test is insensitive to normal amounts.

(5) *Specificity.*—Not specific, as porphobilinogen and certain drugs give false positives; alkaline urine gives higher values than acidic urines.

b.   Ehrlich's Aldehyde Test for Urobilinogen.—

(1) *Theory.*—Classical test for measuring urobilinogen in the urine. Ehrlich's reagent, *p*-dimethylaminobenzaldehyde, reacts with urobilinogen, or any similar molecule having pyrrole rings, to form a red-colored complex.

(2) *Method.—*

(a)   Place 10 ml urine in a test tube.
(b)   Add 1 ml of Ehrlich's reagent (2% *p*-dimethylaminobenzaldehyde in 50% hydrochloric acid); mix.
(c)   Let stand for 5 min.

(3) *Interpretation.*—Negative test: no development of red color. Positive test: urobilinogen or any other Ehrlich's reactive-compounds give a distinct red color.

(4) *Sensitivity.*—Same as urobilistix.

(5) *Specificity.*—Not a specific test for urobilinogen, since other Ehrlich's reactive-compounds give positive tests.

7.   Hematuria or Occult Blood—Hemastix.—

a.   Hemastix (Orthotoluidine Test).—This test is for intact red cells (hematuria) or hemoglobin (hemoglobinuria) in the urine.

(1) *Theory.*—The reaction is based on the peroxidase activity of hemoglobin. Hemoglobin reduces peroxide, liberating oxygen, which oxidizes orthotoluidine from a colorless dye to a blue dye.

$$\text{orthotoluidine} + H_2O_2 \xrightarrow[\text{peroxidase activity}]{\text{Hb}} \text{orthotoluidine} + H_2O$$
$$\text{(colorless)} \qquad\qquad\qquad\qquad\qquad\qquad \text{(blue)}$$

(2) *Method.—*

(a)   Dip test area of strip into well-mixed urine.
(b)   Drain excess urine.
(c)   Wait 30 sec and compare test area of strip to the color chart.

(3) *Interpretation.*—Negative test: no color development, test area remains buff color. Positive test: blue color develops; different shades of blue indicate small, moderate or large amounts of hemoglobin.

(4) *Sensitivity.*—The test is more sensitive for free hemoglobin than for intact cells. Orthotoluidine test will pick up presence of hemoglobin at a level of about 0–0.0003 mg/ml of urine.

(5) *Specificity.*—The test is not specific as hemastix reacts with intact red cells, free hemoglobin and myoglobin. False positive tests may be due to peroxidase from white blood cells. False negative tests may be due to ascorbic acid, which inhibits color reaction. The occult blood screening test should also be accompanied by a microscopic examination of the sediment to detect presence of red cells. In hematuria the sediment is positive for red cells. In pure hemoglobinuria no red cells are seen in the sediment.

b. **Benzidine Test.—**

(1) *Theory.*—The peroxidase activity of hemoglobin catalyzes the oxidation of colorless, reduced benzidine by hydrogen peroxide to oxidized blue benzidine.

$$\text{benzidine} + H_2O_2 \xrightarrow[\text{peroxidase activity}]{Hb} \text{benzidine} + H_2O$$
$$\text{(colorless)} \qquad\qquad\qquad\qquad\qquad\qquad \text{(blue)}$$

(2) *Method.*—

(a) Place into a test tube 1 ml of urine; dilute with 5 ml of distilled water. Add, in the following order

(b) 1 ml of 1% benzidine dihydrochloride

(c) 1 ml of 3% hydrogen peroxide

(d) 1 ml of 1% sodium acetate

(3) *Interpretation.*—Negative test: no color development. Positive test: a blue color develops in presence of blood. The rapidity of color development depends on amount of blood present. Color develops within 1–10 sec.

(4) *Sensitivity.*—Same as for orthotoluidine test.

(5) *Specificity.*—Same as for orthotoluidine test.

NOTE: The orthotoluidine test is recommended because of benzidine's carcinogenic effects.

8. **Phenylketonuria or PKU Disease —Phenistix.—**The PKU disease is caused by hereditary lack of the enzyme phenylalanine hydroxylase. The enzyme is necessary for the conversion of the amino acid phenylalanine to the amino acid tyrosine. The type of disease is known as an "inborn error of metabolism."

   Normal Reaction —

$$\text{phenylalanine} \xrightarrow[\text{hydroxylase}]{\text{phenylalanine}} \text{tyrosine}$$

In the absence of the enzyme, phenylalanine accumulates in the blood and is converted to phenylpyruvic acid, which is excreted in the urine.

PKU Disease —

$$\text{phenylalanine} \xrightarrow[\text{phenylalanine hydroxylase}]{\text{in absence of}} \text{phenylpyruvic acid}$$

As phenylalanine in the diet accumulates in the blood, it causes brain damage and mental retardation. If the individual lacks this enzyme as an infant, he/she must be kept on a phenylalanine-free diet for the first 5 years of life. During this time the nervous system is completing its development. After this period the person could be returned to a normal diet as the nervous system is no longer affected by the phenylalanine.

Testing of the urine for phenylpyruvic acid is a way of detecting PKU disease; the test is done with phenistix.

(1) *Theory.*—The ferric ion, impregnated in the phenistix, reacts with phenylpyruvic acid to form a bluish-grey to grey-green color.

(2) *Method.*—

(a) Dip test area of strip into the urine or press strip onto a wet diaper.
(b) Compare test area of strip to color chart within 30 sec.

(3) *Interpretation.*—Negative test: no color development within 30 sec. Positive test: color changes from grey to grey-green within 30 sec.

(4) *Sensitivity.*—Test is sensitive for phenylpyruvic acid as low as 5–10 mg/100 ml urine.

(5) *Specificity.*—The test is nonspecific, as several substances give false positive results. *p*-Hydroxyphenylpyruvic acid, normally present in the urine, gives a fleeting color reaction which fades within a few seconds.

9. **Combination "Stix" Tests.**—The combination "stix" tests screen the urine for the following substances:

Uristix	Protein, glucose
Ketodiastix	Ketones, glucose
Combistix	pH, protein, glucose
Hemacombistix	pH, protein, glucose, occult blood
Labstix	pH, protein, glucose, ketones, occult blood
Bililabstix	pH, protein, glucose, ketones, bilirubin, occult blood
Multistix	pH, protein, glucose, ketones, bilirubin, occult blood, urobilinogen
N-multistix	All of the above, plus nitrite test for bacteriuria

Note again: Not all of these tests are performed as part of the "routine urinalysis." The chemical tests done as routine are for protein, glucose and acetone. Some laboratories include bile as a routine determination. The PKU is done on all newborn infants. The other tests discussed in this section are usually considered ancillary to the basic tests.

PROGRAMMED QUESTIONS

Cover answers with a piece of paper. Answers appear at end of questions.

(1) What is the major reagent of the Clini-test tablet and Benedict's solution?
(a) Sulfosalicylic acid
(b) Cupric sulfate
(c) Peroxidase
(d) Cuprous oxide

(2) What is the proper order for the metabolic breakdown of hemoglobin?
(a) Urobilinogen, bilirubin, urobilin
(b) Urobilin, urobilinogen, bilirubin
(c) Bilirubin, urobilinogen, urobilin
(d) Bilirubin, urobilin, urobilinogen

(3) Which reagent "stix" test will give a false positive reaction if the urine pH has changed?
(a) Albustix
(b) Ketostix
(c) Clinistix
(d) Phenistix

(4) What reagent will demonstrate the presence of metabolites formed due to the incomplete metabolism of fats?
(a) Cyanide
(b) Orthotoluidine
(c) Sulfosalicylic acid
(d) Nitroferricyanide

(5) Which substance can demonstrate occult blood in the urine?
(a) Hemoglobin
(b) p-Dimethylaminobenzaldehyde
(c) Orthotoluidine
(d) Phenylpyruvic acid

(6) What is the metabolic defect in PKU disease?
(a) Presence of tyrosine
(b) Absence of phenylalanine
(c) Presence of p-hydroxyphenylpyruvic acid
(d) Absence of phenylalanine hydroxylase

(7) From the list below, which is the only specific test?
(a) Glucose oxidase
(b) Acetest
(c) Clinitest
(d) Ehrlich's test

(8) With what will the diazo dye of the Ictotest react solely?
(a) Porphobilinogen
(b) Bilirubin
(c) Glucose
(d) Urobilinogen

(9) What does brownish discoloration indicate on reagent test strips?
(a) Strips have been subjected to refrigeration
(b) Strips have already been used in a urinalysis screening test
(c) Loss of reactivity
(d) None of the above

(10) What reagent will demonstrate protein in the urine?
(a) Rothera's reagent
(b) Orthotoluidine
(c) Monoethanolamine
(d) Sulfosalicylic acid

Answers

(1) b		(6) d	
(2) c		(7) a	
(3) a		(8) b	
(4) d		(9) c	
(5) c		(10) d	

14

Complete Routine Urinalysis—Part III

C. Microscopic Examination of the Urinary Sediment

1. **Types of Substances in Urinary Sediment.**—There are four types of substances that appear in the urinary sediment.
   a. Cells ⎫
   b. Casts ⎬ —the formed elements
   c. Crystals
   d. Amorphous deposits

2. **Type and Age of Sample Examined.**—The a.m. sample is best to use, since it is most concentrated. The sample examined should be freshly voided, preferably within 1–2 hr, but no older than 8 hr.

3. **Preparation of the Urinary Sediment.**—

   a. Mix urine well to suspend cells, casts, etc.
   b. Pour 10–12 ml into a conical-tipped centrifuge tube.
   c. Centrifuge at 2000 rpm for 5 min.
   d. Decant supernatant carefully so as not to upset sediment. Pour off supernatant rapidly all at one time. The supernatant fluid that remains on the walls of the tube is sufficient to resuspend the sediment.
   e. Flick bottom of centrifuge tube with finger to resuspend sediment.
   f. Place 1 drop of the unstained sediment on one end of a slide; cover with a cover slip. (Some prefer not using a cover slip.) In the unstained sediment all substances can be identified.
   g. Stained sediment is used by inexperienced technicians to help them identify the formed elements of the sediment. Sternheimer-Malbin stain (S-M stain) is used to stain the sediment. It consists of crystal violet and safranin. The stain is prepared as follows.

Solution I:	Crystal violet	3.0 g
	95% Ethyl alcohol	20.0 ml
	Ammonium oxalate	0.8 g
	Distilled water	80.0 ml

Solution II:	Safranin O	1.0 g
	95% Ethyl alcohol	40.0 ml
	Distilled water	400.0 ml

Mix 3 ml of solution I with 97 ml of solution II; filter. Filter Sternheimer-Malbin stain every few weeks; discard after 3 months. Solutions I and II keep indefinitely.

After removal of 1 drop of unstained sediment from the centrifuge tube, add 1 drop of Sternheimer-Malbin stain to the urinary sediment. Mix stain and sediment. Wait 3 min for cells and casts of the sediment to accept the stain.

h. Place 1 drop of stained sediment on the other end of the slide; cover with a cover slip. Comparison can then be made between stained and unstained sediment.

Lugol's iodine may also be used as a stain.

4. **Microscopic Examination of the Urinary Sediment.**—Examine both stained and unstained sediment under reduced or subdued light. Scan the microscopic fields with low power and then high power to make specific identification of substances. Focus continuously with the fine adjustment.

5. **Types of Tests Performed on Urinary Sediment.**—Both qualitative and semiquantitative tests can be performed.

   a. **Qualitative Tests.**—Observe different kinds of cells, casts and crystals.

   b. **Semiquantitative Tests.**—Count the relative number of different kinds of cells, casts and crystals. To perform a semiquantitative test, examine three random fields. Count the number of cells and casts present, average the results and report. Some laboratories count 10 random fields.

6. **Constituents of Urinary Sediment Examined for Under Low Power.**—

   a. Epithelial cells
   b. Casts
   c. WBC
   d. Crystals
   e. RBC
   f. Cylindroids
   g. Mucus
   h. *T. vaginalis*
   i. *Candida (Monilia) albicans*
   j. Bacteria
   k. Spermatozoa

7. **Constituents of Urinary Sediment Examined for Under High Power.**—

   a. Epithelial cells
   b. Type of casts
   c. WBC (verification)
   d. Crystals (verification)
   e. RBC (verification)

   f. Bacteria

   g. *T. vaginalis* (verification)

   h. *Candida (Monilia) albicans* (verification)

   i. Spermatozoa

8. Constituents of Urinary Sediment Reported/Average LPF.—

   a. Casts

   b. Crystals (just report as present—no quantitation)

   c. Mucus (just report as present—no quantitation)

   d. Epithelial cells

9. Constituents of Urinary Sediment Reported/Average HPF.—

   a. WBC

   b. RBC

   c. Bacteria (few, moderate, many)

   d. *T. vaginalis*

   e. *Candida (Monilia) albicans*

   f. Spermatozoa

10. Cells of the Urinary Sediment (See Fig. 14.1 for Diagrams of the Following).—

   a. Epithelial Cells of the Urinary Tract.—The epithelial cells are sloughed off or desquamated from the inner lining of the tract into the urine as the urine passes. The cells are of various shapes, which are indicative of where the epithelial cells originated.

      From various regions of the kidney nephron, the cells are either simple squamous, cuboidal or columnar epithelium.

      From ureter and bladder, the cells are transitional epithelium, a type of stratified epithelium.

      From urethra, the cells are stratified squamous epithelium.

      Most epithelial cells are of the squamous type and are normally present in moderate amounts in urinary sediments, especially in the female urine due to sloughing of vaginal epithelium.

      Epithelial cells stained with Sternheimer-Malbin stain have dark purple, centrally located nuclei and blue to purple cytoplasm.

   b. Circulating Blood Cells.—In normal urine, blood cells are found in small numbers; high numbers of blood cells indicate abnormalities. How blood cells normally enter the urine is not known. There are more white cells in the urine than red cells; many of them are of urethral or vaginal origin.

      (1) *Erythrocytes.*—Normally, either none or 1–2/2–3 HPF. Red cells increase in the urine during fever and exercise. Increase in red cells in the urine is called hematuria. The hematuria is mainly due to bleeding into the urinary tract, but there are other causes as well (e.g., vaginal contamination during menstruation). The red cells are shiny, round yellow structures in unstained sediment; they stain lavender in color with Sternheimer-Malbin stain.

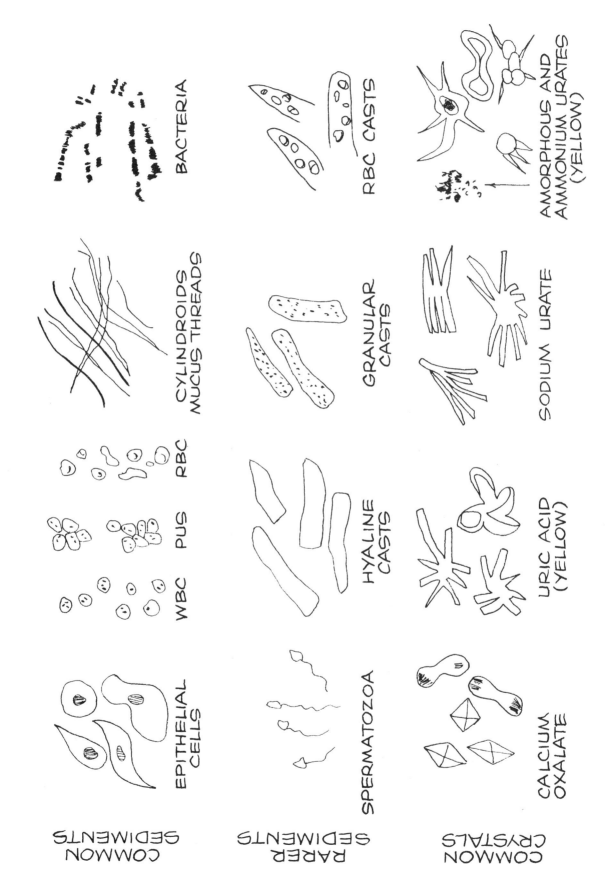

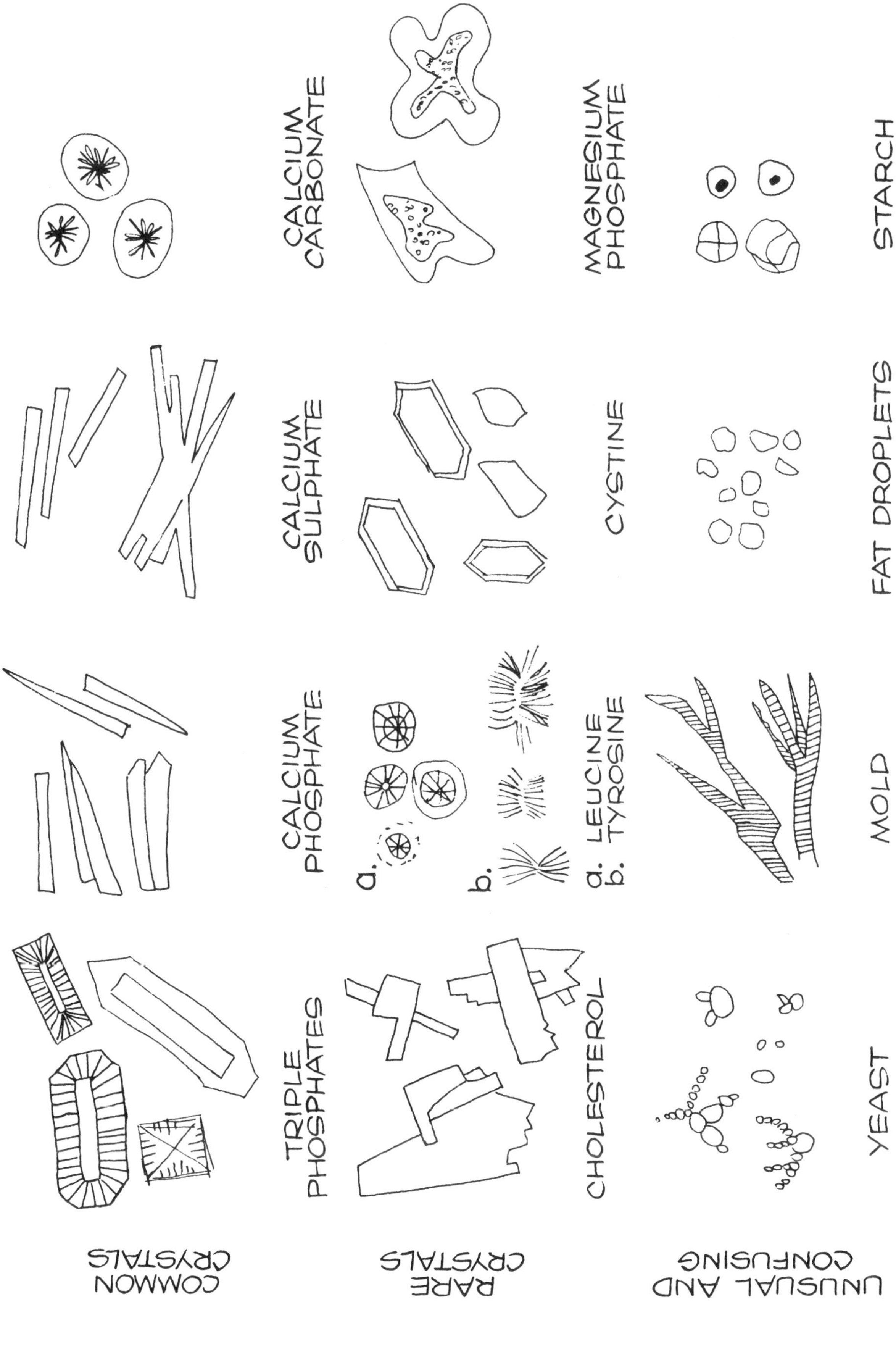

COMMON CRYSTALS

CALCIUM CARBONATE

CALCIUM SULPHATE

CALCIUM PHOSPHATE

TRIPLE PHOSPHATES

RARE CRYSTALS

MAGNESIUM PHOSPHATE

CYSTINE

a. LEUCINE
b. TYROSINE

CHOLESTEROL

UNUSUAL AND CONFUSING

STARCH

FAT DROPLETS

MOLD

YEAST

FIG. 14.1. SOME CONSTITUENTS FOUND IN URINARY SEDIMENT

(2) *Leukocytes.*—White cells in the urine are found normally: occasionally in males and slightly more often in females. White cells increase in the urine during fever and exercise. There is an increased number of white cells seen in all renal diseases and urinary tract infections. The predominant type of white cell is the neutrophil, which can be recognized by its granular nature and lobed nucleus. The leukocytes' cytoplasm stains pink and the nuclei purple with Steinheimer-Malbin stain.

"Glitter cells" are swollen neutrophils which are found in dilute or hypotonic urine. The neutrophilic granules in the cytoplasm shine or glitter. The cells stain light blue to almost colorless.

11. **Casts.**—Urinary casts are precipitated protein in the nephron which becomes molded to the nephron's wall. The casts are formed in lower parts of the nephron. The pieces of cast break off and are washed out into the urine. Casts are cylindrical in shape with parallel side walls and either round or flat ends, and usually with one end appearing to be irregular.

Classification of Casts.—Casts consist of a mucoprotein matrix in which there are granules or organized structures. Casts are classified on the basis of their morphology.

a. **Hyaline or Clear Cast.**—The hyaline cast consists of a matrix of protein, which is transparent in an unstained sediment. To observe hyaline casts in an unstained sediment, reduce the light. On Sternheimer-Malbin staining, the matrix stains pink to purple. Hyaline casts are occasionally found in normal urine and they do not indicate any pathology. Other types of casts described below do indicate renal diseases.

b. **Granular Casts.**—The granular casts, which may be degenerating cellular casts, have either fine or coarse granules. The granules stain purple, while the matrix is pink in Sternheimer-Malbin stain.

c. **Fatty Casts.**—The fatty casts contain highly refractile fat droplets. The fat droplets are unstained, while the matrix stains pink.

d. **Waxy Casts.**—Waxy casts are similar to hyaline casts, but opaque. The waxy casts have curled ends and cracks in the cast.

e. **Cellular Casts.**—In cellular casts, the matrix stains pink, while the cells stain purple-violet.

(1) *Epithelial Cell Cast*
(2) *Leukocyte (Pus) Cast*
(3) *Erythrocyte Cast.*—Unstained, the red cells appear yellow to orange in color.
(4) *Hemoglobin (Blood) Cast.*—Contains hemoglobin from degenerating red cells.

12. **Miscellaneous Substances Found in Urinary Sediments.**—

a. **Cylindroids.**—Cylindroids are long ribbon formations resembling hyaline casts, but longer and with tapered ends which curl. According to some authorities, the cylindroids have the same clinical significance as hyaline casts. Others believe them to be of no significance, and to perhaps be a form of mucus.

b. **Mucus Threads.**—Mucus threads are long thin wavy fibers which taper and branch.

c. **Urinary Tract Infectious Organisms of Both Females and Males.**—

(1) *Trichomonas vaginalis.*—Flagellated protozoa present in the urine due to vaginal contamination. The protozoan causes urethral and bladder infection.

(2) *Candida (Monilia) albicans.*—Yeast in the urine due to vaginal infection. Yeast can be confused with red cells since both are of the same size, but the growing yeast cells bud and adhere together in short chains.

Both are transferred during coitus, and reinfection from male to female or vice versa is possible.

d. **Bacteriuria.**—Pus, clumps of white cells and bacteria. A significant bacteriuria is present if bacteria are $> 10^5$/ml of urine. Bacteriuria is most common in pregnant women and young females. The test for bacteriuria (other than microscopic examination) is microstix. For this test, clean catch urine is necessary. The microstix is dipped into the urine and placed in a sterile plastic bag for 18–24 hr for incubation (at 37°C) of the bacteria. Microstix has three test areas. The first test area is for total bacteria; the second test area is for Gram-negative bacteria, most of which are enteric bacteria. The third test area is the nitrite test. Certain bacteria have the reductase enzyme which reduces nitrate to nitrite.

$$NO_3 \xrightarrow{\text{reductase}} NO_2$$

By comparing the test areas to the color chart, interpretation of the results can be made. A catheterized sample may be used by the bacteriology laboratory to culture and subculture and do sensitivity tests on urinary tract organisms (see *Laboratory Manual of Clinical Bacteriology* in this series).

e. **Spermatozoa.**—Spermatozoa can be present in male and female urine samples.

f. **Artifacts.**—Cotton, hair, fibers, granules of starch or talc. To test for starch, use iodine; starch granules turn blue-black. Starch granules resemble cystine crystals and must be checked.

13. **Urinary Crystals and Amorphous Deposits.**—A variety of crystals is found in normal urine. The types of crystals found depend on the pH of the urine. Crystals are normal in the sediment; unless large in number they generally have no significance. They should be reported as present, but not quantitatively. Many crystals are not present when urine is first voided, but form after the urine cools. The crystallization may be because the urine is supersaturated at cooler temperatures or because change in pH alters the solubilities of these substances. One must recognize commonly occurring crystals in order that the unusual crystals may be distinguished.

a. **Crystals Found in Normal Acid Urine.**—These crystals precipitate out when the urine's pH is acidic. The urate crystals are a result of nucleic acid metabolism.

(1) *Amorphous Urates.*—These are urates of Ca, Mg, K. These crystals are yellow-red, unorganized granules having no specific form or shape. The amorphous urates look like background debris on the slide.

(2) *Sodium Urate.*—These are colorless to yellow crystals, in the form of fans or slender prisms or needles.

(3) *Uric Acid.*—These are yellow to red-brown crystals that have a large variety of shapes (polymorphous). Some are hexagonal plates, others are rhombic plates, wedges or rosettes.

The color of the urate crystals is due to the urobilin.

(4) *Calcium Oxalate.*—These are small, colorless, refractile or shiny, octahedral crystals. They appear as small squares crossed by two diagonal lines. If crystals are viewed from the side they are dumbbell-shaped. The size of these crystals varies greatly. They are of vegetable origin.

(5) *Calcium Sulfate.*—These rare crystals are colorless, long thin needles.

Crystals in acid urine are redissolved on addition of alkali or by warming to 60°C.

The main crystals of acidic urine are the urates.

b. **Crystals Found in Normal Alkaline Urine.**—These crystals precipitate out when the urine's pH is alkaline.

(1) *Amorphous Phosphates.*—This colorless to whitish-pink, fine precipitate looks like background debris on the slide.

(2) *Triple Phosphate.*—This crystal consists of ammonium magnesium phosphate. The crystals are colorless, either 3- or 6-sided prisms or "coffin lids" in shape. They are sometimes feathery or leaf-like in arrangement when in process of dissolving.

(3) *Calcium Phosphate.*—This is a rare colorless crystal, needle-shaped, or needles in a star-shaped pattern.

(4) *Ammonium Biurate.*—These are yellow to brown crystals, spheres or "thornapple" in form. The "thornapple" crystal is a crystal covered with points.

(5) *Calcium Carbonate.*—This crystal is not typical in human urine, unless the patient is on a high vegetable diet. The crystals are colorless granules, spheres or dumbbell-shaped.

Crystals in alkaline urine are redissolved in dilute acids.

The main crystals of alkaline urine are the phosphates.

c. **Crystals Found in Abnormal Urine.**—These crystals precipitate out in acidic urine.

(1) *Cystine.*—The condition is known as cystinuria. The cystinuria is due to a defect in tubular reabsorption of the amino acid. The cystine crystals precipitate out in the urinary tract. The crystals are colorless, flat, hexagonal plates. These crystals are soluble in alkali and in dilute hydrochloric acid.

(2) *Tyrosine.*—Tyrosine crystals are rare except in acute liver failure, when tyrosine is not metabolized. The tyrosine crystals are colorless to yellow needles in bundles or rosettes.

(3) Leucine.—Leucine crystals are yellow spheres with radial and concentric striations or a combination of both.

(4) Cholesterol.—Cholesterol crystals are rare, colorless plates with a notched corner.

(5) Sulfonamide Crystals.—These crystals appear in the urine after administration of sulfa drugs. The crystals are yellow-brown in color, appear as bundles of fine needles or with striations, or round with radial striations. Modern sulfonamide preparations are highly soluble so they rarely precipitate to produce sulfonamide crystals.

PROGRAMMED QUESTIONS

Cover answers with a piece of paper. Answers appear at end of questions.

(1) What is the predominant cell type observed in a urinary sediment of a healthy person?
(a) Leukocytes
(b) Erythrocytes
(c) Epithelial cells
(d) Spermatozoa

(2) Choose from the list below what two substances are stained only by Sternheimer-Malbin stain.
(a) Casts, cells
(b) Cells, crystals
(c) Crystals, casts
(d) Amorphous deposits, crystals

(3) Which cast is opaque and has a curled end?
(a) Fatty
(b) Granular
(c) Blood
(d) Waxy

(4) *Candida albicans* is a _____ infection.
(a) Bacterial
(b) Yeast
(c) Protozoal
(d) Mucus

(5) From the list below, choose two crystals which are found in normal alkaline urine.
(a) Calcium phosphate, calcium sulfate
(b) Amorphous urates, calcium oxalate
(c) Ammonium urate, triple phosphate
(d) Triple phosphate, amorphous urates

(6) How many hours must microstix be incubated before reading the results?
(a) 18–24 hr
(b) 10–12 hr
(c) 36–50 hr
(d) 1–2 hr

(7) From the list below, choose a crystal which is polymorphous in shape.
(a) Sodium urate
(b) Magnesium sulfate
(c) Uric acid
(d) Calcium phosphate

(8) Which crystals have notched corners?
(a) Sulfonamide
(b) Cholesterol
(c) Cystine
(d) Triple phosphate

(9) What cells are usually characteristic of hypotonic urine?
   (a) Glitter cells
   (b) Squamous epithelial cells
   (c) Erythrocytes
   (d) No cells, as cells lyse in such urine

(10) _____ are molds of the nephron walls.
   (a) Crystals
   (b) Proteins
   (c) Sediments
   (d) Casts

Answers

(1) c
(2) a
(3) d
(4) b
(5) c

(6) a
(7) c
(8) b
(9) a
(10) d

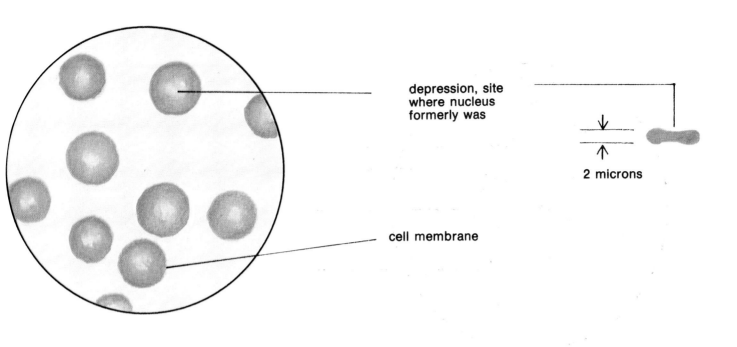

depression, site
where nucleus
formerly was

2 microns

cell membrane

SURFACE VIEW

SIDE VIEW

FIG. 3.7. ERYTHROCYTES—MATURE RED CELLS

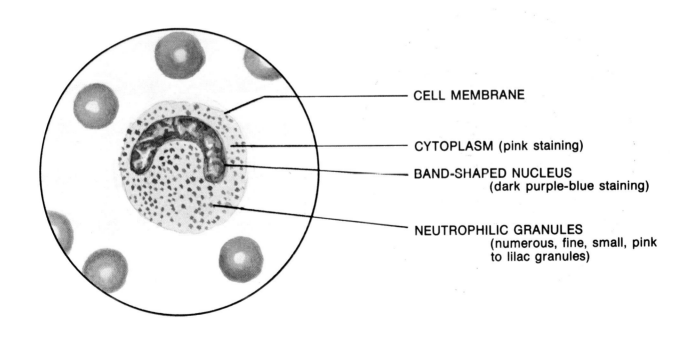

CELL MEMBRANE

CYTOPLASM (pink staining)

BAND-SHAPED NUCLEUS
(dark purple-blue staining)

NEUTROPHILIC GRANULES
(numerous, fine, small, pink
to lilac granules)

FIG. 3.8. BAND OR STAB CELL

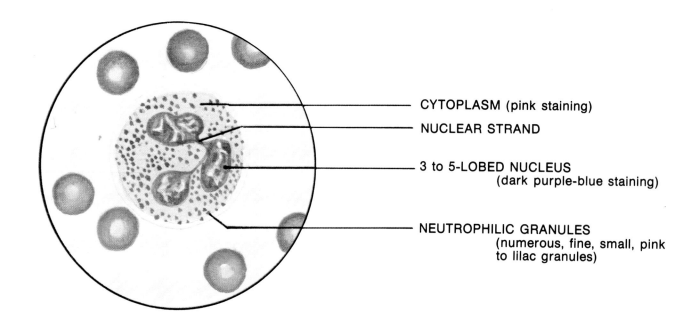

CYTOPLASM (pink staining)

NUCLEAR STRAND

3 to 5-LOBED NUCLEUS
(dark purple-blue staining)

NEUTROPHILIC GRANULES
(numerous, fine, small, pink
to lilac granules)

FIG. 3.9. MATURE NEUTROPHIL(E) OR POLYMORPHONUCLEAR LEUKOCYTE

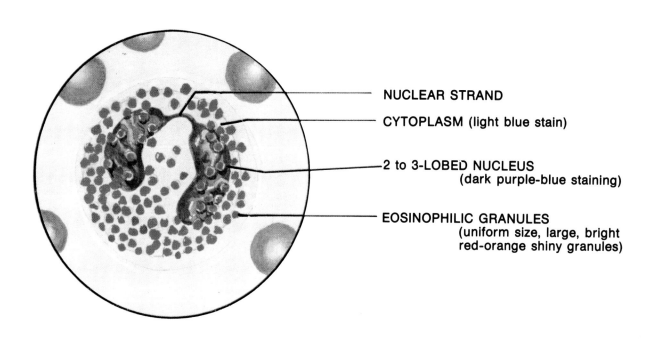

NUCLEAR STRAND

CYTOPLASM (light blue stain)

2 to 3-LOBED NUCLEUS
(dark purple-blue staining)

EOSINOPHILIC GRANULES
(uniform size, large, bright
red-orange shiny granules)

FIG. 3.10. EOSINOPHIL(E)

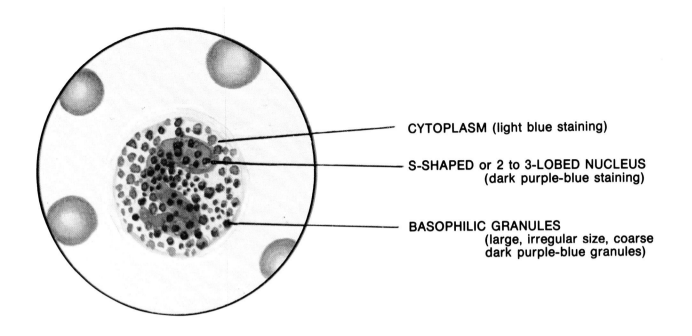

CYTOPLASM (light blue staining)

S-SHAPED or 2 to 3-LOBED NUCLEUS
(dark purple-blue staining)

BASOPHILIC GRANULES
(large, irregular size, coarse
dark purple-blue granules)

FIG. 3.11. BASOPHIL (E)

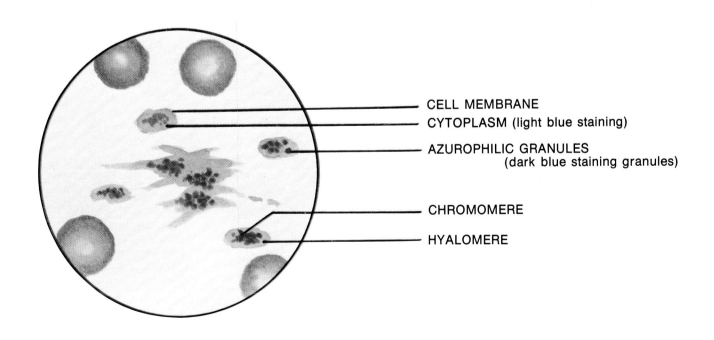

CELL MEMBRANE

CYTOPLASM (light blue staining)

AZUROPHILIC GRANULES
(dark blue staining granules)

CHROMOMERE

HYALOMERE

FIG. 3.12. PLATELETS (THROMBOCYTES)

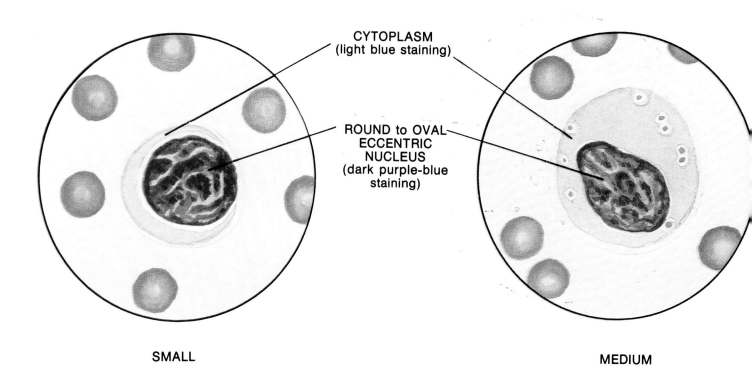

CYTOPLASM
(light blue staining)

ROUND to OVAL
ECCENTRIC
NUCLEUS
(dark purple-blue
staining)

SMALL

MEDIUM

FIG. 3.13. LYMPHOCYTES—SMALL AND MEDIUM

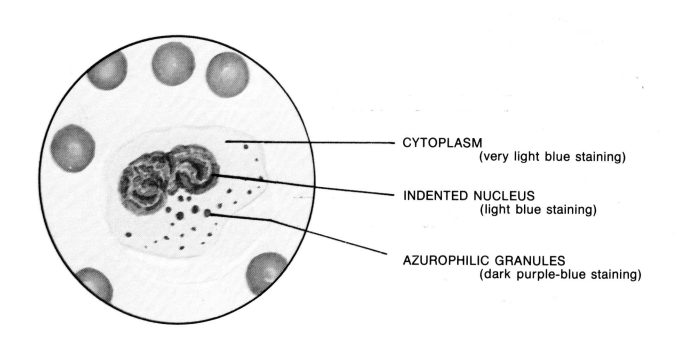

CYTOPLASM
(very light blue staining)

INDENTED NUCLEUS
(light blue staining)

AZUROPHILIC GRANULES
(dark purple-blue staining)

FIG. 3.14. MONOCYTE

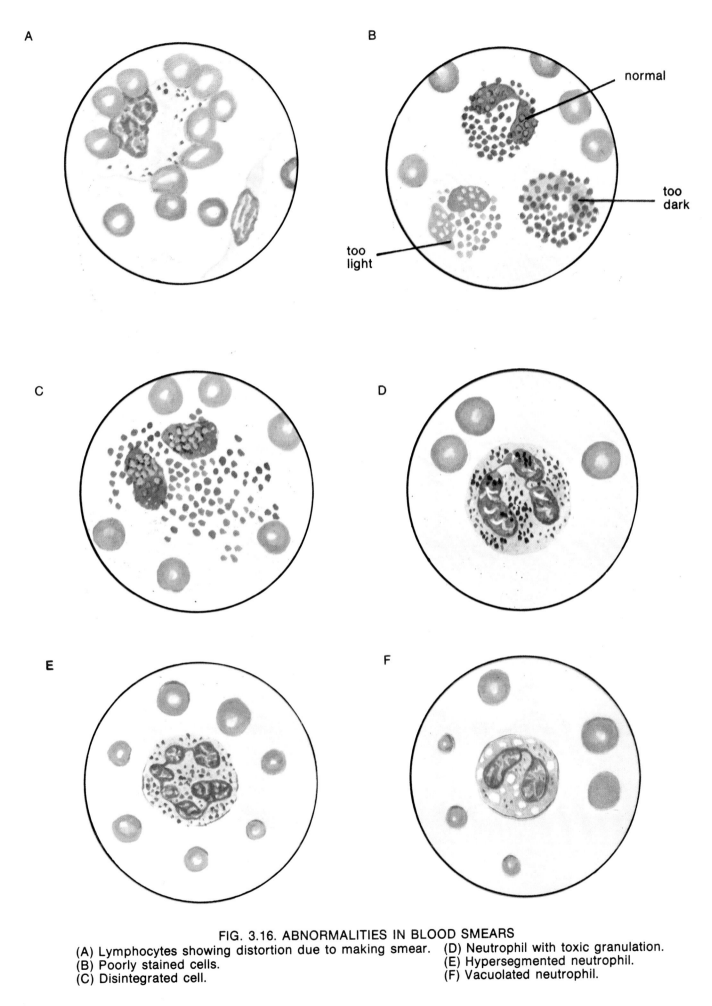

FIG. 3.16. ABNORMALITIES IN BLOOD SMEARS

(A) Lymphocytes showing distortion due to making smear.
(B) Poorly stained cells.
(C) Disintegrated cell.
(D) Neutrophil with toxic granulation.
(E) Hypersegmented neutrophil.
(F) Vacuolated neutrophil.

A

B

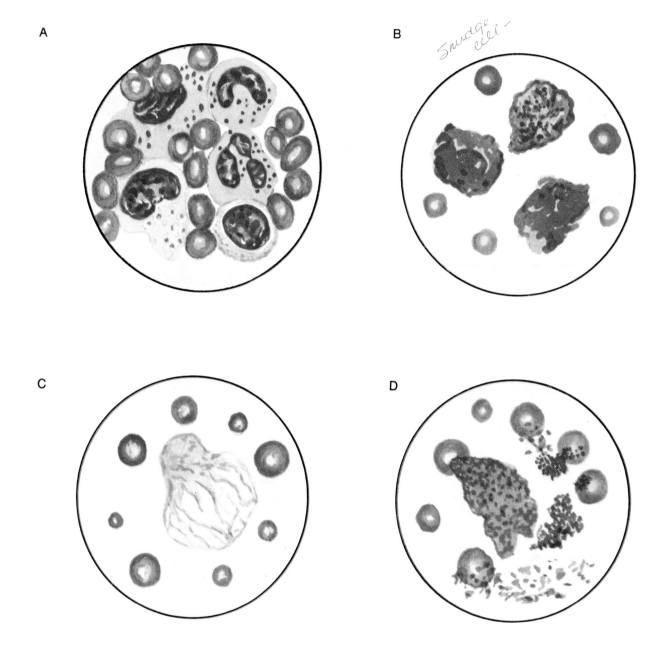

C

D

FIG. 3.17. ABNORMALITIES IN BLOOD SMEARS
(A) White cells at edge of smears.   (C) Basket cell.
(B) Smudge cells.   (D) Precipitated stain.

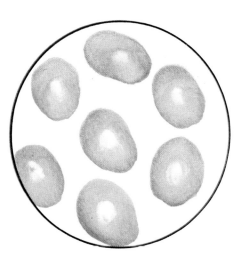

FIG. 9.1. RED CELLS WITH NORMAL
AMOUNT OF
HEMOGLOBIN: CI = 1.0

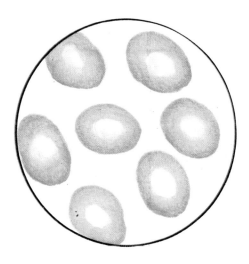

FIG. 9.2. RED CELLS WITH ONE-HALF
THE NORMAL AMOUNT OF
HEMOGLOBIN: CI = 0.5

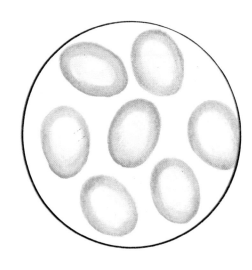

FIG. 9.3. RED CELLS CONTAINING
ONE-TENTH THE NORMAL AMOUNT OF
HEMOGLOBIN: CI = 0.1

Stain: WRIGHT'S

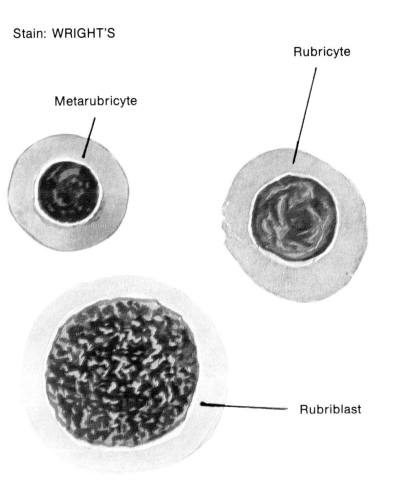

Metarubricyte

Rubricyte

Rubriblast

NUCLEATED RED CELLS

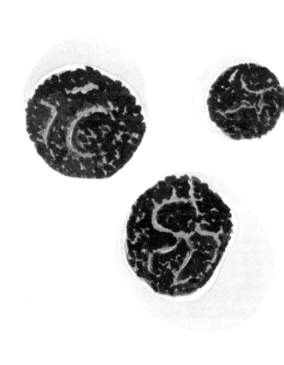

LYMPHOCYTES

FIG. 11.1. COMPARISON OF NUCLEATED RED CELLS AND LYMPHOCYTES

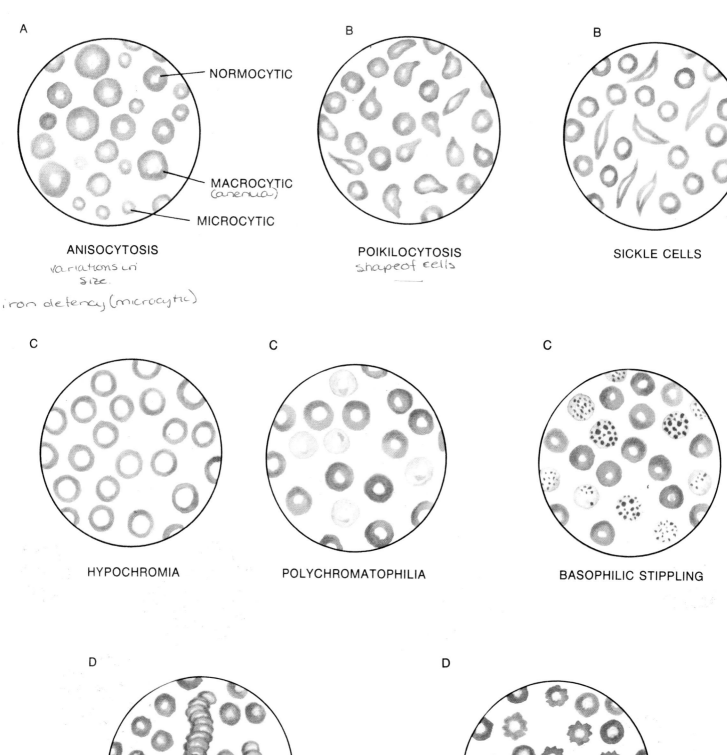

A

NORMOCYTIC

MACROCYTIC
(anemia)

MICROCYTIC

ANISOCYTOSIS

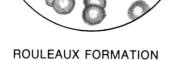

POIKILOCYTOSIS
shape of cells

SICKLE CELLS

HYPOCHROMIA

POLYCHROMATOPHILIA

BASOPHILIC STIPPLING

ROULEAUX FORMATION

CRENATED ERYTHROCYTES

FIG. 11.2. ABNORMAL ERYTHROCYTES

(A) Differences in size.   (C) Differences in content.
(B) Differences in shape.   (D) Miscellaneous differences.